REHABILITATION
OF THE
OLDER PATIENT

A handbook for the multidisciplinary team

Edited by
Amanda J. Squires

London and Sydney
CROOM HELM

First published in 1988 by Croom Helm Ltd
11 New Fetter Lane, London EC4P 4EE

Published in Australia by Croom Helm Australia
44–50 Waterloo Road, North Ryde 2113, New South Wales

ISBN 0 7099 5423 9

British Library Cataloguing in Publication Data

Rehabilitation of the older patient.
1. Old persons. Rehabilitation. Medical
aspects
I. Squires, Amanda   II. Series
618.97
ISBN 0–7099–5423–9

Distributed exclusively in the USA by Sheridan House Inc.
145 Palisade Street, Dobbs Ferry, NY 10522

Typeset in 10/12 pt Times
by Mayhew Typesetting, Bristol
and printed in Great Britain by
St. Edmundsbury Press, Bury St. Edmunds, Suffolk

Contents

Contributors

Penelope Fenn Clark Grad DipPhys MCSP
Superintendent Physiotherapist
Dulwich Hospital North, London

Katherine Coombes DipCOT
Community Occupational Therapist
The Economic Commission, London

Alison Froggatt MA BA AIMSW
Lecturer in Social Work
University of Bradford

James George MB MRCP
Consultant Physician in Geriatric Medicine
Cumberland Infirmary, Carlisle

Rosemary E. Gravell BMed Sci MCST
Chief Speech Therapist
Riverside Health Authority

Linda Haldane MCSP
Superintendent Physiotherapist for Care of the Elderly
St Stephens Hospital, London

Jean Hall DipCOT MBAOT
Principal Occupational Therapist, Training and Development
Officer
London Borough of Hillingdon

Thelma Harvey BA MCSP
Community Physiotherapist
London Borough of Islington

Marion Judd MNZSP MCSP
Community Physiotherapist
Islington Health Authority

Judith Kemp MSc SRCh
Chief Chiropodist
City and Hackney Health Authority

Adrienne Little BA MPhil
Principal Clinical Psychologist
Camberwell Health Authority, London

Rosemary Oddy Grad DipPhys MCSP
Superintendent Physiotherapist
Carlton Hayes Hospital, Leicestershire

Amanda Squires Grad DipPhys MCSP MSc
District Physiotherapist
Waltham Forest Health Authority

Cameron G. Swift PhD FRCP
Professor of Health Care of the Elderly
Kings College School of Medicine and Dentistry
and Dulwich Hospital, London

Madeline Taylor DipCOT
formerly Head Occupational Therapist (Psychiatry)
Lewisham and North Southwark Health Authority, London

Linda Thomas RGN
Editor
Geriatric Nursing and Home Care

Patricia Wardle MCSP DipED
Minister of United Reformed Church, London

Lindsay Winterton MCSP
Superintendent Physiotherapist
Princess Louise Hopsital, London

John Young MB MRCP
Consultant Physician in Geriatric Medicine
St Lukes Hospital, Bradford

Acknowledgements

The authors and editor would like to thank the following individuals:

Chapter 3: Eli Garlant DipCOT SROT and Joanna Moon MCSP SRP for their comments and advice; Lyn Gregory for typing.

Chapter 4: K. Clark for library assistance; L. Holliman for assistance with Appendix I; M. Thompson for typing.

Chapter 6: K. Clark for library assistance; M. Thompson for typing.

Chapter 9: Dr J. Chatterjee, Dr P.L. Chin and Mrs M. Robson for assistance.

Chapter 10: Colleagues from St Luke's Hospital, Bradford who allowed the author to share their work for a short period; Primrose Wright and Jan Burrows for helpful advice; Elaine Goldsbrough for typing.

Chapter 12: Colleagues of the Physiotherapy and Occupational Therapy Departments for advice and support.

Chapter 13: Carol Easteal and Brian Dockerill for supplying photographs; Mike Heasman for the scale model; John Morgan for the chart and drawing (Table 13.1 and Figure 13.4).

Preface

Attitudes to rehabilitation of older patients, particularly in departments specialising in care of the elderly, have become increasingly positive in recent years. A growing number of professionals see the speciality as a necessary career experience and this needs encouragement if the professions are to be prepared for the increasing number of older people who will require help from their members.

The purpose of this book is to bring together the skills and experience of experts in several fields of rehabilitation of the older patient to provide a primer for those needing the knowledge of how to manage the older patient in whatever environment or speciality they present. Readers will be able to enhance their own knowledge gained in a variety of fields and play an immediate part in the team.

Currently many of the judgements made by team members are based on 'experience' or 'intuition', seldom available to the student or newly-qualified person. The multiple facets of management of the older patient may quickly overwhelm and deter the unprepared. The 'team' concept may also be new and links between disciplines and the service each provides can easily confuse the new participant and be a potential minefield. We hope, in this book, to have clarified some of these areas. Two particular topics have, however, not been covered in this book. Details of the organisation of health care, including structure, planning, financing and private care, together with the core contribution of the Primary Health Care Team, have not been included. This is because of wide international variation and alternative available literature.

1

Disease and Disability in the Elderly — Prospects for Intervention

Cameron G. Swift

INTRODUCTION

In spite of much progress, the provision of health care for older people is still widely perceived as a problem, rather than as a stimulating challenge awaiting professional application. Overriding considerations of a rapidly expanding dependent elderly population confronting a fixed system of supply and demand for services, have often led to negative and defensive strategies, which stifle innovation and engender professional rejection of the old and their particular health-care needs.

This chapter will attempt to argue the case against such an approach by tracing the principles which have emerged in the evolution of modern geriatric medicine, together with some of the achievements which have been documented. In this way, appropriate, tangible and positive objectives can be identified which open the way to further progress and without which the vulnerable older members of our society will be the continued targets of considerable disservice. While resource provision is obviously a critical factor, the writer's personal view is that many problems have their origin in concept rather than in quantity, in professional practice rather than in plant. The philosophy underlying this volume is the potential for intervention and treatment as distinct from accommodation and 'care', and it is therefore appropriate to begin with a consideration of objectives.

PRINCIPLES

The emergence of old-age medicine as a defined discipline has been accompanied by the recognition of a composite foundation of certain principles, which include the following:

(i) 'Normal' ageing may be compatible with good health.

(ii) Care and skill in the diagnosis of disease in the elderly are not only appropriate but critical to proper management.

(iii) Assessment of function — physical, mental and social — should always occur in parallel with medical diagnosis and treatment.

(iv) Difficulties in diagnosis and assessment commonly occur because of atypical disease presentation and concurrent disorders.

(v) Organised professional teamwork and proper linkage to other informal and formal agencies are essential at all stages.

(vi) The skills of problem-identification and multidisciplinary 'management by objective' are at least as important as those of traditional diagnosis and prescription.

(vii) The capacity of older people to recover from illness and regain complete or partial independence should not be underestimated.

(viii) The organisation of care should be so structured as to eliminate delay, minimise personal disruption and ensure continuity of information and professional contact.

HISTORICAL PROGRESS

The extent to which these interdependent concepts have been developed and given organised expression has largely governed the 'success' or otherwise of health-care services for the elderly in any locality. Since the pioneering work of Marjory Warren (1948) in the 1930s and 1940s the track record of many departments under the supervision of clinicians specialising wholly or partly in the care of the elderly, has been well documented, especially within the framework of the United Kingdom's National Health Service (NHS) and its district general hospitals. The cardinal achievement has been the shift in emphasis from custodial care to successful therapeutic intervention — an investment in the capacity of the older person to respond to treatment and in the willingness of a caring community network to stay involved in helping him or her with the practical problems of independent daily living.

DEFINING AND CALCULATING THE NEED

Quantitative measurement of this process has been somewhat crude, predominantly analysis of hospital activity (such as waiting times, numbers of admissions and discharges and duration of stay) rather than results for patients themselves and there is still an urgent need to derive usable, clinically-orientated measures of therapeutic performance in evaluating the care of older people. Standards have, nevertheless, been set, especially for elimination of delay in intervention, access to high-quality care and treatment, and prospects for successful restoration to community living after significant illness; against these the performance and efficiency of future initiatives should be compared.

These standards should also govern the type and amount of resource provision if the challenges posed by demographic trends are to be properly addressed. The latter have been reviewed by Muir Gray (1985). In essence, a major increase in the absolute numbers of elderly people, especially the very elderly (75+ years), is currently in progress, particularly in developed countries, as a result of the sharp reduction in infant mortality during the twentieth century. The male:female ratio in old age is broadly about 1:3 because of the protective effects of oestrogens against atheroma and the hitherto more hazardous lifestyle pursued by men (including the World Wars, smoking, alcohol, reckless driving and homicide).

In determining service provision, other demographic characteristics, such as the relative numbers of supporting adults, migration patterns of elderly people and their families, changes in family structure, economic status and availability of adequate housing all require proper scrutiny. In the United Kingdom, for example, large numbers of older people migrate to certain coastal or rural retirement communities, whilst the families of many living in deprived inner city areas have moved away to the suburbs or beyond. It is important to recognise that these factors may influence not only social structure, but also health, and that a corresponding provision of health service resources will therefore be required.

3

INTERRELATIONSHIP OF DISEASE AND DISABILITY IN THE ELDERLY

It is well known that a number of diseases which cause disability become more common with advancing age, although this is clearly not always the case, as for instance in the demyelinating diseases. Examples include cerebrovascular disease, Parkinson's disease, dementia, the commoner forms of arthritis and osteoporosis. In addition, some diseases encountered in the elderly are often at an advanced stage of progress, for example chronic airflow obstruction or ischaemic heart disease. Other conditions, such as normal pressure hydrocephalus and pseudo-gout are more specifically 'old-age disorders'.

Illness and 'function'

All these, together with a reduction in physiological and functional 'reserve' resulting from the normal ageing process, constitute the backcloth against which modern acute and preventative old-age medicine is practised.

The level of function achieved by an older person with one or more such conditions may remain remarkably stable (if suboptimal) for long periods. When, however, an acute intercurrent disease (e.g. an infection) or exacerbation of one of the underlying conditions (e.g. cerebral or myocardial infarction) occurs, the immediate effect on function is frequently dramatic, so that the whole range of disorders presents in the form of a functional or social crisis, with or without clear-cut signs of the acute disease itself.

Successful management of such complex clinical situations requires an immediate response, skilled assessment and highly-organised teamwork if the risk of long-term dependency is to be avoided. It is very difficult, as a rule, to predict in advance the range and scale of problems from an initial presumptive diagnosis. The likelihood that these will be considerable does, however, increase exponentially with age. This is apparent from cohort population studies, such as that of Harris (1971), which showed that over 50 per cent of the total population of Great Britain classed as severely handicapped was aged over 75 (to what extent such handicap is preventable constitutes a challenging question). It is also suggested by analysis of hospital in-patient data, which show an exponential increase with age in the predicted duration of stay from the time of admission to hospital, particularly from the age of 75 and upwards.

ACHIEVEMENTS IN THE DELIVERY OF CARE

Measuring progress in the health care of the elderly will never be easy. Few indicators of 'success' enjoy universal acceptance, and there is at times heated controversy amongst the general public, health and social services professionals, informal carers, administrators and even older people themselves as to what is desirable. While some of this debate may be useful in focusing attention on the needs of the elderly, lack of consensus can also be a major barrier to concerted action, and it is important to identify common objectives.

Developments in the United Kingdom

In the writer's view, it is important to retain an historical perspective. Recognition of the special needs of the elderly sick in the United Kingdom had its initial expression in the Poor-house infirmaries associated with the accumulation in the Poor-houses of many chronically sick, disabled and financially destitute elderly people. These large institutions were characterised as recently as the 1940s and 1950s by massive overcrowding, long durations of stay (average about three years), high patient dependency, long waiting lists for admission, minimal prospects of discharge (except by death), fear in the minds of older people, massive strain on relatives and community resources, superlative basic nursing care and negligible medical input (Thompson 1949). In general, they were conceptually and geographically isolated from the 'mainstream' medical activity concentrated in the voluntary hospitals and the emphasis was on palliation of symptoms and behavioural disturbance as distinct from any targeted therapeutic intervention. Acutely ill old people in the community were perceived as potential 'bed-blockers' and general practitioners therefore had difficulty in persuading medical staff in the 'acute' hospitals to accept them for admission.

Assumption of responsibility for the Poor-house infirmaries by the newly-formed health authorities provided the setting for the pioneers of modern geriatric medicine, such as Marjory Warren and her

5

contemporaries. They applied positive principles of systematic diagnosis, assessment and treatment, and together with their colleagues in the nursing, remedial and social work professions, planned and achieved the successful return of many patients of varying degrees of disability to realistic periods of community life. Many were also removed from the waiting lists for admission.

Under the umbrella of the NHS, these early lessons have been applied to a greater or lesser extent across the health districts of the United Kingdom, with increasing recognition of the eight principles outlined earlier. The value of specialist departments based in mainstream district general hospitals, offering immediate access for medically-ill old people to the full range of diagnostic, assessment, treatment and remedial facilities, and staffed by physicians and professional co-workers with specific accountability for their care, has been set out in several published studies (Hodkinson and Jefferys 1972; Bagnall *et al.* 1977; Evans 1983; Rai *et al.* 1985; Horrocks 1986; Mitchell *et al.* 1987).

Measuring health-care performance

As stated above, the outcome has been measured predominantly in terms of hospital activity. Total numbers of hospital beds per head of elderly population have been dramatically reduced, waiting lists and bed-blockage have been abolished, the throughput of patients has been greatly increased (typically twelve or more patients per bed per year, some 10 to 15 per cent only of beds at any one time being occupied by patients staying in hospital more than six months) and overall average duration of stay reduced to 20 to 30 days. Such departments have been characterised by a clearly-defined role in the acute medical care of the elderly (e.g. responsibility for those over 75), by operational policies promoting continuity of care, by efficient liaison with the community and with other hospital services (usually by means of a central information/liaison office) and by positive policies of rehabilitation and discharge, with well-developed multidisciplinary teamwork (Horrocks 1986).

The contribution to 'community care' made by this hospital-orientated model consists, to some extent, in its accessibility to, and dialogue with, general practitioners, district nurses, informal carers and other community-based agencies. Respite admissions and day hospital activity feature prominently. Other important consequences include the ready recruitment of high-quality professional staff, the obvious scope for training and research, and clear-cut departmental 'identity'.

Viewed in the historical context, it can be argued that clear benefits for patients have been achieved, notably removal of the problems of access to hospital treatment without delay and of the fear of waiting to 'go into hospital to die'. Relatives and other carers retain an involvement, sustained by organised support and the knowledge that rescue in a crisis or planned relief are available without delay. These are important criteria of progress with which few would disagree. They constitute documented evidence of a workable balance between community and hospital care, based on professional commitment within the framework of a defragmented service. Such a framework is critical, since fragmentation of care is a particular hazard faced by the elderly if their multiple or recurring problems are addressed solely by the various agencies of a system-specialised medical service, with disjointed community support, and no planned coordination.

Developments in education

The logical movement of specialist departments into mainstream hospitals has provided the foundation for medical education in the care of the elderly. Organised teaching of undergraduate medical students in this discipline now takes place in all United Kingdom medical schools and, to a varying extent, in many medical schools in the United States, Canada, Australasia and Europe. The number of Academic Departments of Geriatric Medicine or Health Care of the Elderly continues to grow, providing a focus for research into the medicine of old age, the process of ageing and the delivery of care. The involvement of allied professions, including nurses, remedial therapists and social workers, in the formal education of medical students and staff is encouraged and valued in many modern departments. Specific training in the special needs of the elderly is represented to a varying degree in the curricula of these professions themselves.

COMMUNITY CARE

Much of the above discussion has centred on the historical development of hospital-based services. It is well known, however, that the care of the elderly is undertaken predominantly outside hospitals or institutions, although the hospital constitutes a focus of concentrated acute need and high dependency. Since most older people are likely to experience some hospital contact at some stage, the role of hospital care and its relationship to the community is a major determinant of the long-term outcome they obtain. Prospects for community living, however, particularly if there is disability, depend fundamentally on the range of accommodation and services available. These services include primary medical care, community nursing and health visiting, remedial therapy, clinical psychology, chiropody, dental, ophthalmic and audiological services, social work, residential care, home care and day care provision (Horrocks 1986).

An important point is that older people are often unaware themselves of their entitlement, a problem which the voluntary organisation, Age Concern, has sought to address in the publication of its booklet *Your Rights* (Age Concern 1982). Housing may be a critical factor, and its poor standard often reflects the low economic status of many older people, especially in large urban areas. Rehousing at a later stage is often declined by the very elderly, so that forward-looking policies are necessary for the future, while a responsive and flexible approach to adaptations is needed now. Sheltered housing with warden cover is a growth industry, but where such resources are limited there are difficulties in rationalising their use according to need.

Relatives and informal carers continue to constitute the mainstay of community and long-term care, and the importance of the enabling role of health and social services by providing adequate support, advice and relief has already been mentioned and cannot be over-stressed. Rejection by relatives is the exception rather than the rule, and is usually the result of too little support too late. Voluntary bodies, including Age Concern and the Association of Carers, have done much to highlight the importance of the critical contribution of informal carers, for example *Who Cares in Southwark?* (Bonny 1984).

Effective liaison between social service and health service provision is vital for several reasons, but particularly to ensure that scarce community resources are used economically to meet genuine need and that health problems presenting as social crises do not go unrecognised and untreated. The hospital-based social worker, as a member of the multidisciplinary health care of the elderly team, has historically played a vital role in this respect, providing the operational link with residential care, home helps, meals services, day centres, voluntary agencies, housing departments and community care schemes.

The critical challenge ahead is to eliminate fragmentation of care in the community as well as in the hospital. The activities of any one discipline, whether it be medicine, nursing, remedial therapy, social work or voluntary agency, may at best be wasted or at worst harmful, if they are not related to an agreed assessment and planned programme of care involving the other disciplines.

PROSPECTS FOR THE FUTURE

Measuring outcome

Old-age medicine incorporates a shift in emphasis from the reduction of mortality to the prevention of morbidity, a goal which is much more difficult to quantify. What is absolutely clear is the central importance of measuring *function* as a component of well-being or ill health in the elderly, an exercise which has been conspicuously neglected by doctors in the past (and to some extent, the present!). Physiotherapists have led the way in developing and evaluating the relevant techniques and skills and there is much excellent published work. The subject of functional assessment is explored in detail later in this book. Of the many rating scales and 'quality of life indices' so far devised, however, none has found wide enough applicability or acceptance to be used as a single standard measure of outcome or cost-effectiveness by health care providers. From an operational point of view, the ideal index will need to quantify function in terms of daily living activities and to relate this to support provided. It will also need to be reproducible and manageable in the context of repeated measurement, since there is probably no alternative to longitudinal studies. Such studies will also incorporate the currently available health care 'performance indicators' measuring such criteria as time spent in and out of hospital and other institutional settings.

A common error is to deduce the type and quantity of service provision required from single time-point prevalence studies. The assumption is made, for example, that the amount of perceived disability in a community at any one point in time indicates the need for 'support' and 'accommodation', when in fact the need may be for better and earlier intervention. Such an approach fails to recognise that health problems in old age and their functional and social consequences commonly follow an acute, rapidly-changing, recovering and relapsing pattern, a pattern which may be profoundly affected by the availability or otherwise of skilled diagnosis and properly-organised treatment. Well-designed longitudinal studies should be able to determine the impact of such interventions on the quality of life of the older person from initial presentation or iden-tification to the end of the lifespan. Geriatric medicine, properly practised, is predominantly an acute discipline.

Prevention

So far we have concentrated on how health problems are managed and treated when they present, typically as some form of acute crisis or breakdown in function, and have emphasised that the skilfulness or otherwise of such management may profoundly influence the subsequent prospects for independent living of old people and the numbers requiring long-term institutional care. In other words, good treatment of illness in old age has, to some extent, a preventative function.

A common reaction, however, is to say 'if only this particular problem had been dealt with earlier, it might have been much less serious or prevented altogether; irreversible damage might have been averted'. *Primary* prevention in the sense of dealing with the known cause of a condition and so completely preventing its occurrence has been largely, hitherto, an exercise for the medicine of earlier life. Examples would include the common immunisations, elimination of asbestos exposure and perhaps the elimination of tobacco consump-tion. *Secondary* prevention is concerned with the early detection of disease or its precursors in patients who are asymptomatic and consider themselves fit, and constitutes the rationale for screening programmes.

This can be distinguished from *case-finding*, in which established disease and its consequences are present but for a variety of reasons unreported by the sufferer. Case-finding, with a view to earlier diagnosis and the prospect of better results from treatment, has been described as a form of *tertiary* prevention (Williamson 1981).

The concept of universal screening of the elderly (defined by a given chronological age) has met with little favour, not least because of the unrealistic time required of professional staff (whether general practitioners or other professional health visitors) and the apparently low returns achieved in such a blanket approach. Attention has been focused more on attempting to define categories of old people who are arguably at risk of health problems and to target case-finding initiatives at these groups, as in a survey conducted in Aberdeen (Age Concern Research Unit 1983). The latter, expanding an earlier World Health Organisation (WHO) list, selected the very old (>80), the recently widowed, the never married, those living alone, those socially isolated (not necessarily living alone), those without children, those in poor economic circumstances, those recently discharged from hospital, those who have recently changed their dwelling, the divorced/separated and those in social class V (Registrar General's classification). Interestingly, many of these 'conventional' risk factors proved rather inefficient as markers for case-finding. An alternative two-stage approach, based on an initial postal screening questionnaire, followed, where appropriate, by a comprehensive health visitor assessment, was also described (Age Concern Research Unit 1983). This proved somewhat more efficient, and the analysis of findings suggested further economies based on selecting the most discriminating questions identified. The main benefits overall consisted of determining and addressing a number of unmet needs (mainly contact with available services and treatment of active health symptoms). These benefits were clearly demonstrable, and could also be shown to be achievable with feasible changes in doctor, health visitor and district nurse workload. Evidence of longer-term benefit and actual 'prevention', however, remains to be derived.

Work of this kind primarily provides pointers to further research, particularly longitudinal studies. This should preferably be undertaken as a joint initiative with a viable and well-organised hospital-based service whose positive impact in reducing long-term bed occupancy is well attested. There seems little point in embarking on a study of preventative approaches when there is a fundamental deficiency in the ability of services to meet those unmet needs which are so identified. The evidence that episodes of hospitalisation for older people can be significantly reduced by screening programmes is still awaited, while the evidence that long-term institutionalisation can be delayed or prevented by an efficient geriatric medical service linked strongly to primary medical and community services is more than tangible. The opportunities for general practitioners, physicians in geriatric medicine and the professionals with whom they work to combine their respective skills in further research with an accent on prevention are clearly most exciting. Some cautionary points, however, emerge from the projects already undertaken, in particular:

(i) There is a major necessity to refine both markers of need and measures of outcome in the health care of older people. This requires careful research and observation, since our current perception of health and ill-health determinants, however 'logical', may easily be mistaken.

(ii) 'Prevention' may well (in time) result in much benefit to many old people, but there is no guarantee that it will make their health care cheaper. Indeed, available evidence, in so far as it points up major areas of unmet need, suggests that the opposite may be the case. Thus naive planning assumptions about prevention and 'community care' as economical alternatives to current medical practice are seriously ill-founded.

(iii) It follows therefore, that policy-makers and planners should not divert funds wholesale from existing services to new initiatives unless the latter have been thoroughly validated and shown to be of measurable value to the large majority of older people.

(iv) Resources for well-designed local and pilot studies constitute sound initial investment, whilst ensuring that existing services which are working well remain adequately supported and are made more uniformly available.

SUMMARY

Disease and disability go hand-in-hand with increasing frequency, the older the sufferer. For many decades, while medical science has advanced technically, the disabilities of the old have met with a passive and negative acceptance by medical practitioners, health-care providers and many of the population at large. It is now clear, however, that a positive, organised, professional and to some extent specialised, approach to diagnosis, assessment and intervention can have a major and positive impact on the prospects for continued autonomy of a large majority of ill old people, and on the burdens carried by relatives, families and caring communities. The collaboration and coordination of several professionals and other agencies is a central factor in achieving results. Successful models of health care have been developed and described. These require consolidation and wider application. At the same time research into new patterns of intervention with an accent on preventative health care is now a clear requirement. It presents a challenge to the commitment and skill of all those concerned to ensure a better future for older people.

REFERENCES

Age Concern (1982) *Your Rights*. Age Concern, Mitcham, London

Age Concern Research Unit (1983) *Research Perspectives on Ageing, 6; The Elderly at Risk*. Age Concern, Mitcham, London

Bonny, Z. (1984) *Who Cares in Southwark?* Association of Carers, London

Bagnall, W.E., Datta, S.R., Knox, J. and Horrocks, P. (1977) Geriatric Medicine in Hull: A Comprehensive Service. *British Medical Journal, 2*, 102–4

Evans, J.G. (1983) Integration of Geriatric with General Medical Services in Newcastle. *Lancet, i*, 1430–3

Harris, A. (1971) *Handicapped and Impaired in Great Britain*. HMSO, London

Hodkinson, H.M. and Jefferys, P.M. (1972) Making Hospital Geriatrics Work. *British Medical Journal, 4*, 536–9

Horrocks, P. (1986) The Components of a Comprehensive District Health Service for Elderly People — A Personal View. *Age & Ageing, 15*, 321–42

Mitchell, J., Kafetz, K. and Rossiter, B. (1987) Benefits of Effective Hospital Services for Elderly People. *British Medical Journal, 295*, 980–3

Muir Gray, J.A. (1985) Social and Community Aspects of Ageing. In M.S.J. Pathy (ed.), *Principles and Practice of Geriatric Medicine*, Wiley, Chichester

Rai, G.S., Murphy, P. and Pluck, R.A. (1985) Who Should Provide Hospital Care of Elderly People? *Lancet, i*, 683–5

Thompson, A.P. (1949) Problems of Ageing and Chronic Sickness. *British Medical Journal, ii*, 243–50, 300–5

Warren, M. (1948) Care of the Hemiplegic Patient. *Medical Press, 219*, 396–8

Williamson, J. (1981) Screening, Surveillance and Case-finding. In T. Arie (ed.), *Health Care of the Elderly*, Croom Helm, London.

2

Psychological Aspects of Working with Elderly Clients

Adrienne Little

Psychology, the 'science of mental life' (Miller 1962), is the study of behaviour. It is the role of the clinical psychologist to apply this knowledge to clinical populations. Few clinical psychologists work exclusively with elderly clients — in the United Kingdom only 1 in 20 (Garland 1986) — and most of these work in psychiatric settings. The Health Advisory Service (HAS) report (1983) urged psychologists to develop a comprehensive service within the health, voluntary and local authority settings caring for elderly people. Clients from all agencies experience psychological distress and impairment and they, and staff alike, can benefit from psychological input. The profession is responding to this challenge and three recent reports describe the development of psychological services within geriatric medicine (Twining and Chapman 1983; Larner and Leeming 1984; Bennett 1986). Unfortunately, most services for physically ill and disabled elderly patients still do not have a specialist psychologist. Therefore, rather than describe how a psychologist could work in these settings, this chapter considers the psychological dimensions relevant to all professionals working to rehabilitate these clients. In particular we consider:

(i) Our expectations of old age and the way in which they influence ourselves and our clients.
(ii) The psychological changes with age.
(iii) The psychological effects of illness and disability.
(iv) The environment within which we work and its influence upon our clients' behaviour.
(v) The psychological effects of caring for elderly disabled people.

STEREOTYPES OF OLD AGE

Our expectations of old age can influence our perception of our clients and their behaviour. We must examine these critically and ensure they do not harm our work.

Expectations of age — myth or reality?

The recent increase in the absolute and relative numbers of elderly people is well documented. However, working with elderly clients has been a 'Cinderella speciality'. Among clinical psychologists, this field was one of the least popular with trainees (Liddell and Boyle 1980) and less than one-fifth of recently-advertised posts were filled (Garland 1986). This position is mirrored among other professions working with the elderly (Norman 1982). Thankfully this seems to be changing. The development of services for elderly clients has been given a priority in many countries. The recent expansion of posts has generated training opportunities. This should begin to correct students' misperceptions of the field and encourage them to consider careers within it. Professions are establishing special interest groups to promote their work. These clinical developments are supported by academic growth. Specialist professional departments of old-age psychiatry and health care are encouraging research and teaching opportunities for all professions.

The reluctance of professionals to work with elderly clients may reflect a 'gerontophobia' prevalent in Western society (Busse and Blazer 1980). Most people expect old age to be unpleasant — characterised by infirmity, poverty, forgetfulness and loneliness. An American poll (Harris 1975) found that a third of the under-65s regard old age as the worst period of life and most anticipate problems. This negative view of old age is established early in life (Goldmann and Goldmann 1982). It is reflected in jokes about dentures and incontinence. Even elderly people view their contemporaries with distaste. Rabbitt (1981a) found that many over-75s described their peers as 'dull . . . selfish . . . boring'. This may explain the reluctance of many to regard themselves as old. On a political level warnings of the 'rising tide' and the 'expense' of dealing with the 'burden' of old age reinforce the view of dependence.

This stereotyped view of old age has been termed 'ageism', i.e. 'the pejorative image of someone who is old simply because of his or her age' (Hendricks and Hendricks 1977). As a stereotype, we assume that old age inevitably brings these unwelcome changes. These expectations de-individualise and de-humanise elderly people — we assume that they are all the same and are different from the young. How true is this?

The experience of old age differs from the fantasy. Harris (1975) found that most elderly Americans were pleasantly surprised by old age and few experienced the problems anticipated by the young. The position is similar in Europe. A survey of English elderly found that most rated their general health as good and few were lonely. Half could find nothing to dislike in their lives (Hunt 1978).

The evidence highlights the dangers of assuming that all elderly people are the same and exaggerating differences between young and old. People become more, not less, varied as they age — 'age does not eradicate sex, race and class distinctions . . . (but) adds another dimension of social differentiation to these distinctions of middle age' (Bengsten *et al.* 1977). For example, one element of ageism is the assumption that elderly people are economically deprived. In the West, low income is not an inevitable consequence of old age. Almost a quarter of elderly people in the United States do live below the poverty line, but substantial numbers are affluent (Jackson 1985). In Japan the elderly own more financial assets than any other age group (*Economist* 1987). Financial status in old age is determined by financial status in middle age — the poor remain poor and the rich remain rich.

Examination of other elements of ageism points to the same conclusions. Elderly people are individuals, not a homogeneous group, and old age is built upon the framework of earlier life.

We are surrounded by people who belie ageism. In the United Kingdom there is the Queen Mother in her 80s and internationally there are leaders in their 60s and 70s whose stamina and achievements may be the envy of many 'younger' people. Locally, there can be found the elderly lady who fought off muggers or the centenarian who attributes his physical fitness to daily swims. Yet often the media focus on the plight of a minority of elderly rather than celebrate the achievements of old age.

Origins of ageism

If these stereotypes of old age are myths, why do we cling to them?

There are many possible reasons for ageism. Elderly people may be devalued because, with urbanisation and industrialisation, they no longer control key resources, e.g. land (Gutman 1977). The young may shun them — because they remind us of our own mortality (Busse and Blazer 1980) or because of the way they look (Bromley 1978). Physical changes such as hearing loss limit the elderly person's social skill and discourage others from talking to him or her. This withdrawal and avoidance allows us to retain our fantasies about age because it prevents us from getting to know them as people. Professionals see an unrepresentative sample of ill and disabled elderly clients, yet for some their patients are their first contact with old age. This can reinforce prejudices that inevitably age brings disability.

Ageism may persist because our myths influence the way elderly people are treated and behave. When applied to the individual, the myth may become reality.

Effects of ageism

Society's treatment of elderly people can amount to wholesale discrimination on the basis of age. They are excluded from mainstream society in many ways (e.g. enforced retirement) and often segregated with specialist housing and services. Segregation itself reinforces ageism by imposing boundaries between old and young. As a devalued group the elderly suffer deprivation. Their services receive low priority for the allocation of finite resources (Jackson 1985). Professionals joining these services may be deterred by what they perceive as depressing physical work environments (Coren et al. 1987). Services that are available may fail to respond appropriately because they expect so little of the elderly client. Several studies suggest that general practitioners do not recognise illness among their elderly patients (e.g. Williamson et al. 1964), possibly because we associate age with frailty and infirmity ('It's just her age.')

Low expectations may deprive elderly people of opportunities as well as services. Wolfensberger (1980) describes how unrealistically low expectations produce over-protection and deprivation, which in turn may produce disability. Low expectations can become self-fulfilling prophecies (Figure 2.1).

Elderly people may share ageist stereotypes and devalue and

Figure 2.1: Knowing what's best for mother. 'Protection' can mean deprivation. (If instead the family assume that mother *can*, they will encourage her to *do* and give her opportunities to succeed. Mother's achievement encourages the family (including herself) to expect further success.)

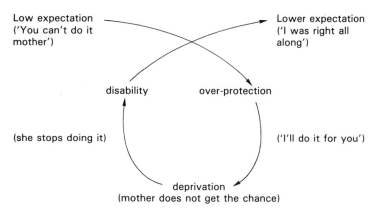

Low expectation ('You can't do it mother')

Lower expectation ('I was right all along')

disability

over-protection

(she stops doing it)

('I'll do it for you')

deprivation
(mother does not get the chance)

deprive themselves. They may fail to recognise illness or seek treatment ('It's just my age') and may hold unrealistically low expectations of their abilities. These expectations can become reality. For example, many elderly people are concerned about their memories (Lowenthal *et al.* 1967) and become more anxious than younger subjects when confronted with memory tests. Eisdorfer *et al.* (1970) showed how this anxiety produces a memory impairment — if the anxiety is reduced then memory performance improves.

Finally, just as society may feel that services for elderly clients do not merit priority for funding, so elderly people may be reluctant to spend their own limited resources (e.g. energy, money) on themselves. An elderly client who feels life is over may not see the point of struggling to walk again or to cook his or her own meals.

PSYCHOLOGICAL CHANGES WITH AGE

Psychologists have studied two types of developmental change in elderly subjects — changes in cognitive ability (e.g. intellect, memory, problem-solving) and in personality and adjustment. Two publications review this literature (Miller 1977; Woods and Britton

1985), and Birren and Schaie (1977) and Botwinick (1978) give detailed reviews of specific areas of study.

What cognitive and personality changes occur with age?

Until the 1960s psychologists emphasised the extent of these developmental changes. Studies comparing old and young suggested that cognitive ability inevitably and progressively declines. Indeed, Wechsler (1958) claimed that intellectual ability peaks in the late 20s or early 30s. Elderly subjects seem more 'anxious', 'depressed' and 'withdrawn' on personality tests. This process of withdrawal was regarded by Cumming and Henry (1961) as part of a successful and desirable adjustment to age. These findings seem to reinforce ageist stereotypes. They are undermined by the substantial numbers of elderly people who carry on working, enrol for courses or join clubs and classes.

Recent work suggests that developmental changes are more complex and subtle. Psychologists now emphasise the continuity of ageing and the variability of developmental changes shown by elderly subjects.

This shift in position came through an awareness of the methodological flaws in earlier studies and development of improved research designs. In the late 1960s Schaie pointed out that age differences reported in earlier studies could be artefacts (Schaie 1967; Baltes 1968). Most of these studies compared samples of old and young, observed a difference and inferred that this represented a developmental change. Thus older subjects do worse because they have declined. The problem of these cross-sectional studies is that differences between groups could result from any number of factors other than age. These factors ('cohort effects') include differences in education, health, exposure to psychologists, etc. To establish a developmental change it is necessary to study samples longitudinally. Even these studies are inconclusive as samples may change for reasons other than ageing, e.g. cultural changes or the impact of repeated testing.

Longitudinal studies of cognitive change do not confirm the picture of inevitable deterioration beginning in middle age. Most report stability of performance, possibly with some decline among very old subjects. Some studies have found improvements with age. There have been very few longitudinal studies of personality change

(Neugarten 1977) — those available emphasise the relative absence of change.

This picture of stability may over-simplify development in old age. Reports from different studies often contradict one another — because they employ different samples and measures. Individuals change at different rates on different measures. Rabbitt (1981b) highlighted the dangers of looking at averages and ignoring individual variability. Within his field of interest (cognitive speed) there are substantial differences between the average reaction times of old and young. However, there are also substantial differences in the scatter of performance. Rabbitt reported that the standard deviation of elderly samples is often considerably larger than that of younger subjects. The old samples seem more varied than the young. Furthermore, the overlap between old and young is considerable. Some elderly subjects are faster than most young and conversely some young subjects are slower than most elderly. Similar variability is found in all fields of study. Gaber (1983), for example, found that his elderly sample showed very different patterns of responses on a standard measure of personality. He identified four different groups — 'normal', 'introverted', 'mature' and 'perturbed' — with very different personality profiles.

A recent study of memory change in old age illustrates this picture of overall stability with individual variability. Part of our expectation is that old age brings memory problems. Many elderly people are concerned about their memory (Lowenthal *et al.* 1967) although most of these worries are unjustified and indicate depression rather than memory impairment (Kahn *et al.* 1975). Generally older subjects do worse than young on tests of learning and memory (Arenberg and Robertson-Tchabo 1977; Craik 1977). The Duke University longitudinal study took a sample of normal elderly Americans (aged between 60 and 94) in 1955 and followed survivors over the next 20 years. McCarty *et al.* (1982) repeatedly assessed these subjects with a battery of memory tests known as the Wechsler Memory Scale (Wechsler 1945). They concluded that 'the amount of change in memory scores after age 60 . . . was generally small'. Cross-sectionally (i.e. comparing their younger and older subjects) education was a more powerful predictor of memory score than age. However, different tests and subjects showed different patterns of change. Tests of non-verbal memory (e.g. copying drawings from memory) showed more decline over time than verbal tests (e.g. remembering a story). They observed considerable variability among their sample. Subjects who survived longer scored better on the tests

to begin with and showed less decline over time (Siegler *et al.* 1982). This finding that cognitive performance and change predict survival is a general one. It suggests that any sudden decline in ability is pathological and should be assessed.

Models of psychological changes

Why do these changes take place and why do some elderly show more change than others? Age itself is not a causal mechanism and cannot explain these changes or individual differences. Chronological age is a measure which indexes other social, biological and historical processes. These processes may be causal and explain psychological change.

'Social age' is determined by the social roles an individual occupies. For example, the 'young' are single, the 'middle-aged' married and the 'elderly' widowed. Schoenfeld (1974) illustrates the relativity of social age — at 48 Pierre Trudeau was 'young' to be prime minister but 'old' to marry a 23-year-old. Changes in social age may produce developmental change (Bengston *et al.* 1977). The social role changes of old age include retirement, bereavement and impending death. Disengagement theory (Cumming and Henry 1961) explains the findings that elderly people are apparently more withdrawn and introverted as reflecting adjustment to social role ageing. Society and the elderly mutually withdraw from one another to prepare for death. Society withdraws by (for example) forced retirement; the elderly person by (for example) becoming more self-absorbed. Others have emphasised the need to come to terms with and review the past as part of preparation for death (Erikson 1963; Butler 1975). Although by no means all elderly people withdraw and contemplate their lives, the changes shown by some may be explained as adjustments to social age.

'Biological age' is not the same as 'social age' although the two covary (e.g. people marry after puberty). Biological ageing is signalled by various physical changes which have a profound impact on the individual's life. Appearances change with wrinkles, grey hair, baldness, etc. A person may become less able to pick up information from the environment as all sensory modalities become less acute. Musculo-skeletal changes impair mobility and interfere with functional independence. Elderly people are prone to developing various illnesses and are generally more disabled by ill-health (Evans 1982).

21

Adjusting to these changes and their implications can be a painful experience. Jones *et al.* (1984) observed that hearing loss is associated with depression and anxiety among 'normal' elderly community residents. Generally, physical health is an important determinant of life satisfaction and illness is associated with depression in elderly samples (Murphy 1982). Physical illness and sensory loss can also impair cognitive functioning (e.g. Bergmann *et al.* 1981) and some suggest that a 'terminal decline' in cognitive performance precedes death (Kleemeier 1962).

Finally, the ageing person has to adjust to dramatic social and cultural changes within the environment as well as the social and biological changes within his or her life. 'Historical age' refers to the effects of cohort or generation. The present elderly generation has had to adjust to profound and continuing environmental change. Born in the era of trams and steam trains, they have learned to use cars and aeroplanes. We have seen that cohort effects may produce significant differences between old and young on psychological measures. This highlights the dangers of applying measures or techniques relevant to younger age groups when working with elderly clients.

Adjusting to social, biological and historical change is fundamental to psychological development. Development is not restricted to childhood but continues throughout life. The experience of adapting to earlier changes influences our responses to present and future experience and we develop skills and strategies to cope with change. Thus the elderly person is more a product of his or her past than his or her old age.

Abnormal ageing and depression

Although our stereotypes exaggerate the psychological effects of ageing, a minority of elderly people do show marked psychological changes. These changes were called 'abnormal ageing' by Miller (1977) to emphasise their significance and unexpectedness. Abnormal ageing refers to the marked and progressive cognitive impairments and emotional and personality changes observed in senile dementia. Norman (1982) describes these changes as 'the death of a personality and mind before the death of a body'. Although dementia is age-related, only approximately one in ten elderly people show evidence of dementia and even then, half of these show only mild impairment

(Kay *et al.* 1964). The progressive, irreversible changes associated with dementia contrast with the sudden cognitive and behavioural changes observed in 'acute confusional states' (Browne 1984). These changes are the direct result of physical illness or medication and are potentially remediable. Finally, depression and anxiety in elderly patients can produce cognitive impairment (Kendrick 1985) although affective and behavioural changes are more pronounced.

These mental health problems increase with age, but most elderly are perfectly normal and show no cognitive or affective impairment. The classic study of the prevalence of psychiatric disorder in the elderly remains that of Kay *et al.* (1964). In this survey of over-65s in Newcastle, almost three-quarters showed no impairment — 11 per cent showed cognitive impairment, a further 11 per cent affective impairment and 4 per cent 'character' (i.e. personality) disorders. However, the prevalence of these impairments rises on acute medical (Bergmann and Eastham 1974) and geriatric (Kay *et al.* 1962) wards. Kay *et al.* (1962) suggest that over half of the patients on geriatric wards show some cognitive impairment and over a third show some affective disturbance. Many patients are admitted to or remain on these wards because they are demented (Stilwell *et al.* 1984). The implication of these studies is that although most elderly people show no impairment, professionals working with physically ill and disabled clients are going to meet many abnormal or depressed elderly patients. These impairments must be acknowledged as significant and need to be assessed to identify their cause and possible treatment. It is not just a matter of age.

PSYCHOLOGICAL EFFECTS OF ILLNESS AND DISABILITY

The high prevalence of psychological dysfunction among samples of physically ill elderly patients is due to several factors. In some cases physical and psychological pathology happen to co-exist, e.g. a depressed lady who fractures her femur. The psychopathology may contribute to the development of illness, e.g. a dementing gentleman who neglects himself because of his failing cognitive ability and becomes malnourished and dehydrated. Psychopathology may be part of the physical illness, e.g. a toxic confusional state. Conversely, physical symptoms may be part of the presentation of psychological dysfunction, e.g. a depressed patient with various non-specific somatic complaints. Finally, some psychological dysfunctions are reactions to physical pathology.

23

Reactions to pathology

Adjusting to the physical changes of normal ageing can be difficult and painful. The impact of pathology is even more marked. Elderly people (like any other age group) vary in their ability to accept illness and disability. Many adjust with admirable facility. Hunt (1978) found that most elderly people living at home experience some pathology but only a minority complain about their health. Factors influencing the individual's reaction to illness include their coping strategies and abilities, the severity and quality of their illness and their social and physical environment.

The process of adjusting to illness and disability has been likened to bereavement (Evans 1982) in that both involve coming to terms with loss.

Some of the losses experienced by an elderly gentleman following a cerebrovascular accident (CVA) are illustrated in Figure 2.2. He and his family have to come to terms with his illness and disability and to accept the losses and implications of this. The effects on their lives are enormous. It is not surprising that this process can produce psychological dysfunctions. These may include behavioural changes (e.g. apathy, irritability), mood disturbance (e.g. anxiety, depression) and cognitive impairment (e.g. forgetfulness).

Figure 2.2: The impact of Mr Smith's cerebrovascular accident (CVA)

Mr Smith's disabilities	Mr Smith's losses	Some of the implications for Mr and Mrs Smith's life
Dysphasia	Skills	He feels a failure
Hemiparesis	Independence	He depends on her
	Health	They have to move to a ground-floor flat
	Appearance	They are worried he may
	Part-time job	have another stroke and die
	Previous hobbies and social life	They become lonely and isolated
		He is very bored and frustrated
		Financial worries
		Sexual difficulties

Similar dysfunctions are characteristic of bereavement. Parkes (1972) suggests that adjusting to the loss of a loved one involves a lengthy process of grief work. He describes various stages. Initially the bereaved person is unable to accept the fact of the loss and experiences intense anxiety and feels 'numb' or 'unreal'. Gradually he may accept it has occurred but still cannot come to terms with it. Denial becomes despair. Eventually he adjusts and is able to reorganise his life. Clients adjusting to pathology may show many of the features of denial and despair. Livingston (1985) describes how their relatives often react similarly with denial or depression.

The same pathology may affect each person differently. In our example Mr Smith was a healthy man who led an active life. His CVA will change this dramatically. Another person (Mr Jones) may find a CVA easier to accept because it has less impact on his life. Mr Jones may have been less active than Mr Smith because of differences in lifestyle or because an earlier illness has already restricted him. Both men have experienced the same event but the significance of their illness is very different for them.

Helping clients to adjust to disability

Difficulties in accepting loss are often accompanied by unrealistic perceptions of ability. Clients (and their families) may deny or minimise disability and become frustrated every time they fail to achieve an impossible goal. Others may exaggerate their impairment and become over-dependent. Clients can only attain their optimum performance if they are helped to accept their losses and view their abilities realistically. Mr Smith's rehabilitation will be more challenging for the therapist than that of Mr Jones. Mr Smith needs support to adjust to his losses before he can maximise his residual abilities.

Lincoln (1983) describes various psychological strategies to help clients accept disability. She advocates:

(i) Setting clear and realistic targets.
(ii) Giving continuous feedback as to progress.
(iii) Rewarding success.
(iv) Involving the client in designing the rehabilitation plan.

Fordyce (1971) emphasises the importance of avoiding failure —

'performance mastery'. To ensure success it may be necessary to break a task down into progressively more difficult components. Clients proceed to more difficult steps only when the preceding ones have been successfully completed. In this way performance is 'shaped'.

Professionals themselves may minimise or exaggerate their clients' disabilities. It is easy to misidentify a client's fear of failure or catastrophic reaction to it as poor compliance or bloody-mindedness. Often professionals focus exclusively upon disability and ignore clients' strengths (abilities, interests, resources). Barrowclough and Fleming (1985, 1986) advocate a 'constructional approach' whereby strengths are used to help meet needs and overcome disability. Strengths are potential assets for rehabilitation. A client's fondness for cigarettes gives the therapist a means of rewarding successful performance. His social skills can be used within his programme to enhance its meaningfulness for him (e.g. walking to his friends in the day room or cooking a snack for them). Be warned — any therapist suggesting using cigarettes (or alcohol, or chocolate with a diabetic patient) as an incentive is likely to provoke heated team debate! It raises important issues of quality versus quantity of life and of individual rights versus institutional restrictions and policies. Many work settings encourage professionals to over-protect their clients and to adopt a 'safety-first policy' (Norman 1980). Rehabilitation necessarily involves a degree of risk. The ways in which these work settings may promote rehabilitation or foster disability are considered next.

PSYCHOLOGICAL EFFECTS OF THE ENVIRONMENT UPON THE ELDERLY CLIENT

A very small minority of European and American elderly people are in institutional care (Grundy and Arie 1984) but most specialist health professionals are hospital-based. The nature of clients' illnesses may necessitate long periods of hospitalisation or residential care.

Exposure to these care environments may itself change clients' behaviour, often in ways which undermine rehabilitation. Institutional environment encompasses three dimensions:

(i) The *physical* environment (space, decor, etc.).
(ii) The *social* environment (frequency and quality of contact between clients or clients and staff, etc.).

(iii) The *organisational structure* and policies which influence the physical and social environments.

Effective rehabilitation may need to begin by examining and changing one or more of these dimensions.

Impact of the environment on behaviour

Most psychologists regard behaviour as a function of the person and his or her environment. One of the first studies to examine this interaction in elderly patients was Cameron's (1941) analysis of nocturnal delirium (agitated, restless behaviour at night). This behaviour results from the type of person (i.e. was restricted to patients with memory impairment) and the environment (i.e. occurred in any dark conditions). Cameron suggested that these patients become disorientated and anxious in the dark because they are unable to remember their surroundings.

Lawton (1982) proposes that disability (or impaired competence) increases the environment's influence on behaviour. He compares 'the relative freedom with which mentally and physically healthy people can live satisfying lives in a variety of both favourable and unfavourable environments' with 'people of lowered competence (who) have difficulty coping with the demands of marginally adequate environments'. A client who is physically disabled, for example, is dependent upon his environment. If the lavatory is inaccessible he becomes effectively incontinent, whereas a physically able client can find and use the most inconvenient toilet.

An implication of Lawton's 'environmental docility hypothesis' is that subtle changes in the environment (which able people might ignore) can have profound effects on the less able. Ford *et al.* (1986) observed that the behaviour of dementing patients is influenced by changes in the level of lighting or background noise. Imagine the effects of incessant (and often competing) television and pop music on these clients. Staff may enjoy this stimulation. However, clients with cognitive impairment (who have difficulty following rapidly changing programmes), hearing loss (who have difficulty interpreting the sounds), blindness (who may not understand where the sounds come from) or a dislike of modern music, may experience it as overwhelming noise. This highlights the importance of tailoring the environment to meet the needs of the client. Staff needs must also be met but in ways which do not undermine the clients. An environment which promotes rehabilitation would allow and encourage the client to be as active and independent as possible. Lindsley (1964) describes the ideal environment as one which optimises and extends clients' functions; but do institutions for elderly clients provide this 'prosthetic environment'?

Studies of institutional environments for the elderly

The classic study is Townsend's (1962) survey of life in residential homes in the United Kingdom. His graphic descriptions detail the misery of residents' lives. He listed several undesirable effects of institutional life upon the elderly including loneliness, loss of privacy, boredom and erosion of identity and self-determination. More recent studies confirm that this picture 'is as accurate today as when Townsend first described it' (Hughes and Wilkin 1980). Similarly, inactivity and isolation are typical among hospital patients. Godlove *et al.* (1982) and Browne (1984) found that patients on geriatric wards spend most of their days sitting doing nothing. There is very little social contact with staff or other patients. Browne (1984) observed that nursing staff spend only 11 per cent of their time talking to patients. Most staff contact relates to physical care. Some patients may enjoy this leisure and solitude; others may not. It is forced on them irrespective of preference.

Unfortunately, the physical care may encourage disability. Baltes *et al.* (1980) observed that nursing home staff often criticise independent behaviour (e.g. a client trying to feed himself) and praise dependence (e.g. the client waiting for staff to feed him). In the short term it is quicker for hard-pressed staff to do something for the client than encourage him to do it himself. Often clients get staff attention only when they are dependent or complain of pain, etc. This reinforces disabled behaviour (Michael 1970). Staff may enjoy clients' dependence which makes them feel 'needed'. Many staff in residential homes prefer the more 'confused' and physically disabled residents whom they find more rewarding (Godlove *et al.* 1980). Some regard their clients as family substitutes and describe them as children. Rules and regulations may also reinforce this over-protective care (Norman 1980). The effect of these staff behaviours is to promote 'excess disabilities'. Brody *et al.* (1971) observed that many elderly hospital patients show handicaps which are greater than their physical and mental disabilities would predict. Developing individualised programmes of care which were tailored to meet the clients' needs and to encourage independence reduced these disabilities and facilitated discharge.

Developing prosthetic environments

Individualised treatments (Brody *et al.* 1971) demand the skills of an expensive and committed multidisciplinary team. Less costly changes can be effective. Grouping chairs in small circles conducive to conversation rather than lined up against the wall promotes social behaviour (Sommer and Ross 1958; Peterson *et al.* 1977). Generally, environmental change is time-consuming and difficult. Staff attitudes and management are fundamental to the success of the endeavour.

King *et al.* (1971) surveyed care in children's homes. They described these environments as client or institutionally orientated depending upon whether care met the needs of the clients or the institution (Figure 2.3).

Figure 2.3: Does the care environment meet the needs of the client or the institution? Adapted from King *et al.* (1971)

Client centred care		Institution centred care
Flexible		Rigid
	e.g. are clients routinely toiletted?	
Individualised		Block treatment
	e.g. do clients sit at the tables waiting for meals?	
Personalised		Depersonalised
	e.g. do clients wear their own clothes?	
Staff and clients are close	e.g. do they eat together?	Social distance

Client-centred care avoids the undesirable effects of institutionalisation. Care orientation influences several dimensions of the physical and social environment. It is easy to imagine how institution-centred care might produce the undesirable effects described by Townsend (1962). For example, many hospitals and residential environments dress their clients from communal hospital stock (generally because of storage and laundry difficulties). Care is depersonalised. This may be convenient for the laundry staff but fails to meet the clients' needs. Clients have to wear clothes and underwear which are not their own and may be labelled 'Hospital Property' (often visibly). This must erode identity. These clothes may not be tailored to their needs and may hinder independence. If clothes fit badly or are hard to fasten the client may be unable to dress or toilet themselves. Clients may be forced to wear colours, etc. they dislike. Their self-determination is eroded. They (or their relatives) may feel embarrassed by their appearance and reluctant to go out, reinforcing boredom and loneliness.

King *et al.* (1971) observed that care orientation was determined by the attitudes, training and management of staff. Other factors (e.g. institutional size, staffing levels and client disability) seemed irrelevant. This suggests that the most effective way to change the institution is to change the attitudes and organisation of staff so that positive care behaviour is built into the regime. These attitudes influence the institution's response to change. Thus to implement a successful personalised clothing scheme it is essential that all staff (professional, care and domestic) believe that clients have a right to wear their own clothes and understand the benefits of this. Without general commitment the scheme will fail. Woods and Cullen (1983) found that the success of attempts to change the care environment depended more on the commitment of service staff than on the perceived benefits for clients. Committed staff actively encouraged unsuccessful programmes whilst less enthusiastic staff discontinued successful changes.

Two recent approaches consider the staff attitudes necessary to create a positive care environment. *Reality orientation* (RO) is a care package developed by Folsom (1968) for elderly disoriented clients. RO describes the social and physical environments which stimulate these clients and reduce their dependence and disorientation. It is not a cure for dementia, but may maximise the dementing client's quality of life. For example, an elderly lady who is disorientated may become distressed (being lost is an unpleasant experience) and behave inappropriately (e.g. may be unable to find or recognise the toilet and so become incontinent). RO would provide the care environment to minimise these effects of disorientation. All staff would use every opportunity to reassure her of who and where she is. Physically, the toilet would be conveniently located and clearly labelled. Staff would train her to find the toilet herself by using environmental clues (e.g. the colour of the door, signs, landmarks, etc.) rather than toilet or pad her routinely. Fundamental to this package are basic staff attitudes. Holden and Woods (1982) describe these as allowing the elderly person:

(i) Individuality as an adult.
(ii) Dignity.
iii) Self-respect.
(iv) Choice.
(v) Independence.

Wolfensberger (1980) similarly emphasises respect, dignity, choice and age-appropriateness as fundamentals of good care. *Normalisation* describes principles for the planning and running of services for devalued clients. These are widely used by services for the mentally handicapped on both sides of the Atlantic. As the elderly are devalued these principles may be relevant here as well. Normalisation encourages professionals to empathise with their clients and imagine the impact of care. The goal of the service is viewed as helping clients regain value — by using valued means to enable them to lead culturally valued lives. Sadly, services for devalued client groups may be devalued themselves. How many 'geriatric' wards are sited in decrepit buildings while 'high technology' specialisms are housed in modern purpose-built facilities? Services may reinforce their clients' devaluation. It is socially valued to share a house with a few friends and have your own bedroom. It is not valued to share a dormitory every night with 30 other people whom you do not choose to live with. It is socially valued to travel by car to a pub. Travelling on a minibus labelled for the handicapped to go to a labelled specialist luncheon club marks clients as 'different' and segregates and devalues them.

Normalised services rehabilitate clients by helping them participate in the ordinary community. These principles challenge many traditional assumptions of 'good care'. They imply that good services require fundamental changes in society's attitude to disability.

Care environment within the client's home

The studies discussed relate to the elderly institutionalised client but their findings apply to the elderly client living at home. Poor architectural design, over-protective relatives, inflexible daily routines, etc. can promote disability at home as in hospital. The elderly lady cared for in her bedroom may be as isolated and bored as her contemporary in hospital. In both settings the care environment may need changing if rehabilitation is to be achieved and maintained.

THE PSYCHOLOGICAL EFFECTS OF CARING FOR ELDERLY DISABLED CLIENTS

Caring for and working with this client group can produce significant psychological stress.

'Informal carers'

Contrary to myth, families do care. Most elderly disabled people are cared for at home, generally by female relatives (Jones and Vetter 1985). These 'informal carers' have been described as 'the hidden patients' (Fengler and Goodrich 1979). Most studies have examined the impact of caring for dementing relatives. This may be more stressful than looking after a physically disabled relative but, in both cases, carers experience considerable burden and strain (Gilleard *et al.* 1984a; Livingston 1985). Carers are confronted with an enormous range of problems during their 'daily grind' (Gilhooly 1984). Gilleard *et al.* (1981) identified five different types of problems presented by dementing relatives — dependence, disturbance, disability, demand and wandering. Very similar problems were experienced by carers of patients recently admitted to a geriatric unit (Sanford 1975). Some problems seem particularly difficult to cope with. Sanford's sample of carers found sleep disturbance and impaired mobility the hardest to tolerate. Gilleard *et al.* (1982, 1984b) found carers seemed more stressed by their relatives' demands upon them (e.g. being unable to leave them alone) than by their dependence. Greene *et al.* (1982) found that carers were most upset by their dementing relatives' mood disturbance and apathetic inactivity. Given this range of demands, it is not surprising that so many carers report anxiety and depression.

Other factors influence the psychological impact of caring. The children of elderly clients experience more strain than do spouses (Gilleard *et al.* 1984b) although they may be more successful carers in the sense of preventing admission to hospital. Generally, children are fitter and better able to cope with the physical demands of care than an elderly spouse. However, they tend to have demands to balance (e.g. families, work) (Fengler and Goodrich 1979). Indeed, some 'children' are elderly themselves. The quality of the relationship between the carer and relative earlier in life is also important (Isaacs *et al.* 1972; Gilhooly 1984). Bergmann (1979) describes how maladaptive relationships between carers and relatives develop from lifelong patterns. The 'fallen tyrant', for example, describes a dominant and powerful member of the family who has lost his former means of control through disability. No longer able to coerce his relatives by physical aggression he may develop other ways of manipulating the family.

Carers may cope with their burden in various ways. Some secure help from family, friends or formal services. This seems to relieve the burden for carers of the physically disabled (Fengler and Goodrich 1979; Zarit *et al.* 1980) but carers of dementing relatives may receive less benefit (Gilleard *et al.* 1984b). One important area of need from services is for information — carers are often struggling with unclear or incorrect ideas about their relatives' illness and prognosis. Given that many react initially to the illness with denial (Livingston 1985) this information may need repetition. The work of voluntary organisations such as the Association of Carers and the Alzheimer's Disease Society have made a considerable contribution in this area. Gilhooly (1984) describes how many carers adjust to their burden by reconstructing it in their own minds. They may remind themselves that 'it could be worse' or 'it's not that bad' or may concentrate on the good aspects of their situation ('she's happy here with me'). Increasingly, professionals are appreciating the importance of 'supporting these supporters'. Carers have needs and unless these are met they will not be able to provide high-quality care. There is little point in struggling to rehabilitate and discharge a patient from hospital if the family are unable to cope at home. It is as important to be realistic about the family's resources as those of the client.

Professional carers

The professional equivalent of the burden and strain experienced by families may be 'burnout'. This describes a state of disillusionment and exhaustion typical among the 'helping professions'. It has been described in professionals working with the elderly (Quattrochi-Tubin *et al.* 1983). The syndrome includes a range of physical (e.g. fatigue, minor ailments), behavioural (e.g. spending less time at work or with clients) and emotional (e.g. boredom, guilt, hopelessness) changes (McConnell 1982). These changes are the result of struggling to meet overwhelming demands with inadequate resources. Edelwich and Brodsky (1980) describe four stages in the process of burnout — enthusiasm, stagnation, frustration, apathy — whereby the ideals of the enthusiastic newcomer are progressively destroyed. Burnout may be contagious. Disillusioned staff have very low expectations of themselves and their clients. If they feel there is no point trying they devalue their clients and deprive them of opportunities. We have seen how unrealistically low expectations can produce disability. These staff may dictate the institutional milieu which may then promote disability. New staff can be subjected to peer pressure to conform to this or be 'selected-out' (Orford 1982).

Whilst all caring professionals are susceptible to burnout those working with elderly mentally or physically infirm clients may be particularly vulnerable. With these clients there is often no cure. Progress can be painfully slow and achievements seem very limited. This may be frustrating to those used to a faster pace of work (Coren *et al.* 1987). A therapist and client may become disillusioned yet have achieved a great deal by preventing further disability or slowing down the rate of decline. The picture is not hopeless as burnout can be prevented and remedied (Squires and Livesley 1984). It is important that managers and new staff are alerted to burnout from the beginning. The solution demands an approach to rehabilitation which benefits both therapist and client. This involves setting realistic, clear goals and monitoring performance. Ideally goals should be achievable within a few days. In this way the client and therapist experience regular success and have continuous feedback on effectiveness. Progressively more stringent criteria of success can be set as rehabilitation progresses. As well as goal-setting, it is important for staff to set limits on their work and to share their feelings about their clients with one another.

SUMMARY

The psychological dimensions of ageing are complex and affect client, carer and professional alike. An elderly client's behaviour is

Figure 2.4: Incontinence: a complex problem in an elderly in-patient

Expectations: 'Old people get like that — there's nothing we can do'

'Causes'	INCONTINENCE	*'Effects'*
Psychological e.g. he is unable to remember where the toilet is		*Client* e.g. feels embarrassed and uncomfortable and may be prone to infections which make the problem worse. He may cut down on fluids and become dehydrated
Physical e.g. his arthritis limits mobility		
Social environment e.g. staff do not have time to train patients to use the toilet and commode them instead		*Family* e.g. also feel embarrassed and are reluctant to take him for outings in case of accidents
Physical environment e.g. he has just moved to a new ward		*Staff* e.g. label him as 'incontinent' but they are 'dealing' with the problem by regular commoding

affected by many factors — his expectations of age, his adjustment to various processes of ageing, his physical health and his social and physical environment. His behaviour will influence in turn his carers and professional supporters. As an example, incontinence (Figure 2.4) is often the result of a complex interaction between physical, psychological and environmental influences (Hodge 1984). It influences the feelings and behaviour of both clients and carers. Underlying these influences are the powerful devaluing stereotypes of age.

The implication of this analysis for rehabilitation of the elderly client is the importance of flexibility. In particular:

(i) Laying aside personal prejudices about age.
(ii) Analysing the client as an individual and developing plans tailored to his particular needs.
(iii) Developing a coherent multidisciplinary approach to assessment and rehabilitation.

'The elderly' are people who happen to have reached a particular age. They are not a group apart and there are no magical skills required to work with them. Rather the challenge for the team is to tailor their professional and social skills to take account of age. This is demanding — but rewarding.

REFERENCES

Arenberg, D. and Robertson-Tchabo, E.A. (1977) Learning and Aging. In J.E. Birren and K.W. Schaie (eds.), *Handbook of the Psychology of Aging*. Van Nostrand Reinhold, New York

Baltes, M.M. (1968) Longitudinal and cross-sectional sequences in the study of age and generational effects. *Human Development, 11*, 145–71

Baltes, M.M., Burgess, R.L. and Stewart, R.B. (1980) Independence and dependence in self-care behaviours in nursing home residents: An operant-observational study. *International Journal of Behavioural Development, 3*, 489–500

Barrowclough, C. and Fleming, I. (1985) *Goal Planning with Elderly People: How to Make Plans to Meet an Individual's Needs: A Manual of Instruction*. Manchester University Press, Manchester

Barrowclough, C. and Fleming, I. (1986) Training direct care staff in goal planning with elderly people. *Behavioural Psychotherapy, 14*, 192–209

Bengston, V.L., Kassachau, P.L. and Ragan, P.K. (1977) The impact of social structure on aging individuals. In J.E. Birren and K.W. Schaie (eds.), *Handbook of the Psychology of Aging*. Van Nostrand Reinhold, New York

Bennett, P. (1986) Developing acute geriatric services: some ideas from the front line. *Clinical Psychology Forum, 3*, 7–10

Bergmann, K. (1979) How to keep the family supportive. *Geriatric Medicine*, 53–7

Bergmann, K. and Eastham, E.J. (1974) Psychogeriatric ascertainment and assessment for treatment in an acute medical ward setting. *Age and Ageing, 3*, 174–88

Bergmann, K., Britton, P.G., Hall, E.H. and Blessed, G. (1981) The relationship of ageing, physical ill-health, brain damage and affective disorder. In W.M. Beattie (ed.), *Ageing: A Challenge to Science and Society (Volume 2)*. Oxford University Press, Oxford

Birren, J.E. and Schaie, K.W. (1977) *Handbook of the Psychology of Aging*. Van Nostrand Reinhold, New York

Botwinick, J. (1978) *Ageing and Behaviour*. Springer, New York

Brody, E.M., Cole, C., Moss, M. and Silverman, H.A. (1971) Excess disabilities of mentally impaired aged: impact of individualised treatment. *Gerontologist, 11*, 124–33

Bromley, D.B. (1978) Approaches to the study of personality changes in adult life and old age. In A.D. Isaacs and F. Post (eds.), *Studies in Geriatric Psychiatry*. Wiley, Chichester

Browne, K. (1984) Confusion in the Elderly. *Nursing, 2*, (24), 698–705

Busse, E.W. and Blazer, D.G. (1980) *Handbook of Geriatric Psychiatry*. Van Nostrand Reinhold, New York

Butler, R.N. (1975) *Why Survive?: Being Old in America*. Harper & Row, New York

Cameron, D.E. (1941) Studies in senile nocturnal delirium. *Psychiatric Quarterly, 15*, 47–53

Coren, A., Andreassi, M., Blood, H. and Kent, B. (1987) Factors related to physical therapy students' decisions to work with elderly patients.

Physical Therapy, 67, (1), 60–5

Craik, F.I.M. (1977) Age differences in human memory. In J.E. Birren and K.W. Schaie (eds), *Handbook of the Psychology of Aging*. Van Nostrand Reinhold, New York

Cumming, E. and Henry, W. (1961) *Growing Old: The Process of Disengagement*. Basic Books, New York

Economist (1987) Granny Power. 17 January 13–14

Edelwich, J. and Brodsky, A. (1980) *Burnout: Stages of Disillusionment in the Helping Professions*. Human Sciences Press, London

Eisdorfer, C., Nowlin, J. and Wilkie, F. (1970) Improvement of learning in the aged by modification of autonomic nervous system activity. *Science, 197*, 1327–9

Erikson, E.H. (1963) *Childhood and Society*. Norton, New York

Evans, J.G. (1982) The psychiatric aspects of physical disease. In R. Levy and F. Post (eds), *The Psychiatry of Late Life*. Blackwell, Oxford

Fengler, A.P. and Goodrich, N. (1979) Wives of elderly disabled men: the hidden patients. *Gerontologist, 19*, 175–83

Folsom, J.C. (1968) Reality orientation for the elderly mental patient. *Journal of Geriatric Psychiatry, 1*, 291–307

Ford, M., Fox, J., Fitch, S. and Donovan, A. (1986) Light in the darkness *Nursing Times*, 7 January, 26–9

Fordyce, W.E. (1971) Psychological assessment and management. In F.M. Krusen, F.J. Kottke and P.M. Ellwood (eds) *Handbook of Physical Medicine and Rehabilitation*. Saunders, New York

Gaber, L. (1983) Activity/Disengagement revisited: Personality types in the aged. *British Journal of Psychiatry, 143*, 490–7

Garland, J. (1986) Promise or performance? Clinical psychology's contribution to the well being of older people in Britain. *Psychology Special Interest Group for the Elderly, 21*, 12–17

Gilhooly, M.L.M. (1984) The social dimensions of senile dementia. In I. Hanley and J. Hodge (eds), *Psychological Approaches to the Care of the Elderly*. Croom Helm, London

Gilleard, C.J., Watt, G. and Boyd, W.D. (1981) Problems of caring for the elderly mentally infirm at home. Paper presented at the 12th International Congress of Gerontology, July, Hamburg

Gilleard, C.J., Boyd, W.D. and Watt, G. (1982) Problems in caring for the elderly mentally infirm at home. *Archives of Gerontology and Geriatrics, 1*, 151–8

Gilleard, C.J., Belford, H., Gilleard, E., Whittick, J.E. and Gledhill, K. (1984a) Emotional distress amongst the supporters of the elderly mentally infirm. *British Journal of Psychiatry, 145*, 172–7

Gilleard, C.J., Gilleard, E., Gledhill, K. and Whittick, J.E. (1984b) Caring for the elderly mentally infirm at home: A survey of the supporters. *Journal of Epidemiology and Community Health, 38*, 319–25

Godlove, C., Dunn, G. and Wright, H. (1980) Caring for old people in New York and London: The 'nurses' aide' interviews. *Journal of the Royal Society of Medicine, 73*, 713–23

Godlove, C., Richard, L. and Rodwell, G. (1982) *Time for Action: an Observation Study of Elderly People in Four Different Care Environments*. Joint

Unit for Social Services Research, University of Sheffield

Goldmann, R. and Goldmann, J. (1982) *Childrens' Sexual Thinking*. Routledge & Kegan Paul, London

Greene, J.G., Smith, R., Gardiner, M. and Timbury, G.C. (1982) Measuring behavioural disturbance of elderly demented patients in the community and its effects on relatives: A factor analytic study. *Age and Ageing, 11*, 38–43

Grundy, E. and Arie, T. (1984) Institutionalization and the elderly: International comparisons. *Age and Ageing, 13*, 129–37

Gutmann, D. (1977) The cross-cultural perspective: Notes toward a comparative psychology of aging. In J.E. Birren and K.W. Schaie (eds), *Handbook of the Psychology of Aging*. Van Nostrand Reinhold, New York

Harris, L. (1975) *The Myth and Reality of Aging in America*. National Council on the Aging, Washington, DC

Health Advisory Service (1983) *The Rising Tide: Developing Services for Mental Illness in Old Age*. NHS Health Advisory Service, Surrey

Hendricks, J. and Hendricks, C.D. (1977) Ageism and common stereotypes. In J. Hendricks and C.D. Hendricks (eds), *Aging in Mass Society*. Winthrop, Mass

Hodge, J. (1984) Towards a behavioural analysis of dementia. In I. Hanley and J. Hodge (eds) *Psychological Approaches to the Care of the Elderly*. Croom Helm, London

Holden, U.P. and Woods, R.T. (1982) *Reality Orientation: Psychological Approaches to the 'Confused' Elderly*. Churchill Livingstone, Edinburgh

Hughes, B. and Wilkin, D. (1980) *Residential Care of the Elderly: A Review of the Literature*. University of Manchester Research Report, Manchester

Hunt, A. (1978) *The Elderly at Home: A Study of People Aged 65 and Over Living in the Community in England in 1976*. HMSO, London

Isaacs, B., Livingstone, M. and Neville, Y. (1972) *Survival of the Unfittest: A Study of Geriatric Patients in Glasgow*. Routledge & Kegan Paul, London

Jackson, P.M. (1985) Economics of an aging population. *Journal of Epidemiology and Community Health, 39*, 97–101

Jones, D.A., Victor, C.R. and Vetter, N.J. (1984) Hearing difficulty and its psychological implications for the elderly. *Journal of Epidemiology and Community Health, 38*, 75–8

Jones, D.A. and Vetter, N.J. (1985) Formal and informal support received by carers of elderly dependants. *British Medical Journal, 291*, 7 September, 643–5

Kahn, R.L., Zarit, S.H., Hilbert, N.M. and Niederehe, G. (1975) Memory complaint and impairment in the aged: The effect of depression and altered brain function. *Archives of General Psychiatry, 32*, 1569–73

Kay, D.W.K., Beamish, P. and Roth, M. (1962) Some medical and social characteristics of elderly people under state care. *Sociological Research Monographs of University of Keele, 5*, 173–93

—————— , (1964) Old age mental disorders in Newcastle-upon-Tyne: Part 1: A study of prevalence. *British Journal of Psychiatry, 110*, 146–58

Kendrick, D.C. (1985) *Kendrick Cognitive Tests for the Elderly*. NFER-Nelson, Windsor

King, R.D., Raynes, N.V. and Tizard, J. (1971) *Patterns of Residential Care: Sociological Studies in Institutions for Handicapped Children*. Routledge &

Kegan Paul, London

Kleemeier, R.W. (1962) Intellectual change in the senium. *Proceedings of the Social Statistical Section of the American Statistical Association*, 290–5

Larner, S.L. and Leeming, J.T. (1984) The work of a clinical psychologist in the care of the elderly. *Age and Ageing, 13*, 29–33

Lawton, M.P. (1982) Competence, environmental press, and the adaptation of older people. In M.P. Lawton, P.G. Windley and T.O. Byerts (eds), *Aging and the Environment: Theoretical Approaches*. Springer, New York

Liddell, A. and Boyle, M. (1980) Characteristics of applicants to the MSc in Clinical Psychology at NELP. *Newsletter of the Clinical Division of the British Psychological Society, 30*, 20–5

Lincoln, N. (1983) Physical handicap. In A. Liddell (ed.), *The Practice of Clinical Psychology in Great Britain*. Wiley, Chichester

Lindsley, O.R. (1964) Geriatric behavioural prosthetics. In R. Kastenbaum (ed.), *New Thoughts on Old Age*. Springer, New York

Livingston, M.G. (1985) Families who Care. *British Medical Journal, 291*, 5 October, 919–20

Lowenthal, M.F., Bissette, G.G., Buehler, J.A., Pierce, R.C., Robinson, B.C. and Iner, M.L. (1967) *Aging and Mental Disorder in San Francisco*. Jossey-Bass, San Francisco

McCarty, S.M., Siegler, I.C. and Logue, P.E. (1982) Cross-sectional and longitudinal patterns of three Wechsler Memory Scale subtests. *Journal of Gerontology, 37*, (2), 169–75

McConnell, E.A. (1982) *Burnout in the Nursing Profession: Coping Strategies, Causes and Costs*. Mosby, St Louis, Missouri

Michael, J.L. (1970) Rehabilitation. In C. Neuringer and J. Michael (eds.), *Behaviour Modification in Clinical Psychology*. Appleton Century Crofts, New York

Miller, E. (1977) *Abnormal Ageing: The Psychology of Senile and Presenile Dementia*. Wiley, Chichester

Miller, G.A. (1962) *Psychology the Science of Mental Life*. Penguin, Harmondsworth

Murphy, E. (1982) Social origins of depression in old age. *British Journal of Psychiatry, 141*, 135–42

Neugarten, B.L. (1977) Personality and Aging. In J.E. Birren and K.W. Schaie (eds.), *Handbook of the Psychology of Aging*, Van Nostrand Reinhold, New York

Norman, A. (1980) *Rights and Risk*. NCCOP, London

——— (1982) *Mental Illness in Old Age: Meeting the Challenge*. CPA, London

Orford, J. (1982) Institutional climates. In J. Hall (ed.), *Psychology for Nurses and Health Visitors*. Macmillan Press, London

Parkes, C.M. (1972) *Bereavement: Studies of Grief in Adult Life*. Tavistock, London

Peterson, R.F., Knapp, T.J., Rosen, J.C. and Pither, B.F. (1977) The effects of furniture arrangement on the behaviour of geriatric patients. *Behaviour Therapy, 8*, 464–7

Quattrochi-Tubin, S., Jones, J.W. and Breedlove, V. (1983) The burnout syndrome in geriatric counselors and service workers. *Activities, Adaptations and Ageing, 3,* (1), 65–76

Rabbitt, P. (1981a) Talking to the Old. *New Society,* 22 January, 140–1
—— (1981b) Cognitive psychology needs models for changes in performance with old age. In J. Long and A. Baddeley (eds.), *Attention and Performance IX.* Lawrence Erlbaum Associates, Hillsdale

Sanford, J.R.A. (1975) Tolerance of debility in elderly dependants by supporters at home: its significance for hospital practice. *British Medical Journal, 3,* 23 August, 471–3

Schaie, K.W. (1967) Age changes and age differences. *Gerontologist, 7,* 128–32

Schoenfeld, A.E.D. (1974) Translations in gerontology — from lab to life: Utilizing information. *American Psychology, 29,* 796–801

Siegler, I.C., McCarty, S.M. and Logue, P.E. (1982) Wechsler Memory Scale scores, selective attrition and distance from death. *Journal of Gerontology, 37,* (2), 176–81

Sommer, R. and Ross, H. (1958) Social interaction on a geriatric ward. *International Journal of Social Psychiatry, 4,* 128–33

Squires, A. and Livesley, B. (1984) Beware of burnout. *Psysiotherapy, 70,* 6, 235–8

Stilwell, J.A., Hassall, C. and Rose, S. (1984) Changing demands made by senile dementia on the National Health Service. *Journal of Epidemiology and Community Health, 38,* 131–3

Townsend, P. (1962) *The Last Refuge.* Routledge & Kegan Paul, London

Twining, C. and Chapman, J. (1983) The clinical psychologists's input to the geriatric team. *Geriatric Medicine,* January, 41–2

Wechsler, D. (1945) A standardised memory scale for clinical use. *Journal of Psychology, 19,* 87–95
—— (1958) *The Measurement and Appraisal of Adult Intelligence.* Williams & Wilkins, Baltimore, Maryland

Williamson, J., Stokoe, I.H., Gray, S., Fisher, M., Smith, A., McGhee, A. and Stephenson, E. (1964) Old people at home, their unreported needs. *Lancet, 1,* 1117–20

Wolfensberger, W. (1980) A brief overview of the principle of normalization. In R.J. Flynn and K.E. Nitsch (eds.), *Normalization, Social Integration and Community Services.* University Park Press, Baltimore, Maryland

Woods, P.A. and Cullen, C. (1983) Determinants of staff behaviour in long-term care. *Behavioural Psychotherapy, 11,* 4–17

Woods, R.T. and Britton, P.G. (1985) *Clinical Psychology with the Elderly.* Croom Helm, London

Zarit, S.H., Reever, K.E. and Bach-Peterson, J. (1980) Relatives of the impaired elderly: Correlates of feelings of burden. *Gerontologist, 20,* 649–55

3

Communication Problems with Elderly People

Rosemary E. Gravell

It is probably safe to say that anyone who works with elderly people will, at some time, be placed in the position of attempting to communicate with someone who has a communication difficulty. The ability to communicate is essential if a person, of any age, is to remain able to take part in life as a social being. As people age their communicative abilities alter, and these 'normal' differences (not necessarily deficits) must be appreciated if there is to be effective interaction between older persons and their carers — be they lay or professional. Furthermore, increasing age brings with it an increased risk of suffering from a specific communication disorder, which may not only be due to medical conditions (such as cerebrovascular accident or Parkinsonism) but may have a social cause, as in the case of institutionalisation.

Lubinski (1981) nicely summed up the importance of this when she wrote: 'The ability to communicate, either verbally or non-verbally, is the single most important skill older people need to remain valued and contributing members of their surroundings.'

It seems appropriate, in order to provide a framework into which to set specific disorders of communication, to consider briefly the process of normal communication.

WHAT IS COMMUNICATION?

Communication is 'the transmission of a message through some type of conventionalised code' (Lubinski 1978/9). It is thus a psychological interaction between two or more people, and depends on the behaviours and skills of both or all participants. However, it

Figure 3.1: Communication chain. Breakdown at any point along the chain may result in a communication disorder

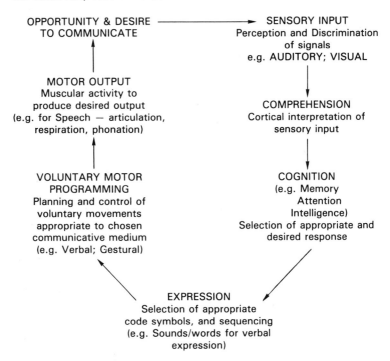

is not restricted to the verbal medium, although this is obviously the primary method which is used whenever possible. Non-verbal communication can add to verbally transmitted messages, or can — if for some reason verbal communication is impossible — become the chosen means.

Verbal communication

The abilities that are necessary if an individual is to be able to communicate effectively via the verbal medium are outlined in Figure 3.1. If there is a break in this 'chain' at any point, difficulty or disorder may result, which may necessitate the use of another medium — either instead of, or to supplement, the verbal.

Verbal communication refers to both spoken and written

Figure 3.2: The brain: lateral view of the left hemisphere

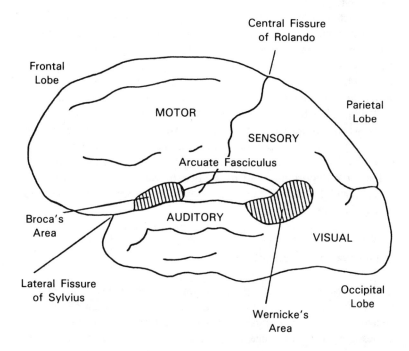

language, and in either case will depend for reception on intact sensory ability. Spoken language obviously depends on hearing, and written language on vision (or touch, e.g. in the case of Braille). Sensory input is then decoded by association areas of the cortex.

Language appears to be a function of the dominant cerebral hemisphere of the brain, which in 90 per cent of people is the left. In the case of auditory input Wernicke's area (Figure 3.2) on the posterior part of the superior temporal gyri is crucial to the process of understanding, that is the interpretation of the incoming sensory impulses. Cognition and language are inextricably linked; and such abilities as attention, memory, and reasoning are critical to communication (verbal or non-verbal).

Association fibres link Wernicke's area to an area located on the lowest part of the precentral gyrus, again in the dominant hemisphere, which is known as Broca's area (Figure 3.2). This site is important to the process of expression, and is implicated, for example, in the ability to select and sequence sounds and words appropriately.

The actual transmission of the message will depend on the ability to programme voluntary motor activity, and finally to perform those necessary movements. In the case of speech these would involve the muscles of articulation, respiration and phonation. Written output would obviously utilise the muscles of the arm and hand. For both verbal and written output postural stability will be important.

This brief outline is far from complete, but does provide a basis from which to discuss what happens when verbal communication fails. However it is important to mention the fact that communication may also break down as a result of psychosocial factors, and that without the opportunity and motivation to want to communicate the process will be halted. Such factors will influence both verbal and non-verbal communication.

Non-verbal communication

It has been stated that verbal communication is usual given the necessary skills, abilities and conditions. However certain non-verbal behaviours are used alongside verbal expression, in order to transmit a message. Tone of voice can, for example, convey the speaker's emotional state — and may even override the spoken content, as in the person who professes contentment through gritted teeth! Intonation will communicate the speaker's intent — whether a question or a statement has been made, or that a conversation is being closed, for instance.

Facial expression and body language may be conscious or unconscious ways of conveying information; while frequently signs or gestures are deliberately employed to support or replace the need for a verbal message. It is worth, at this point, drawing attention to the fact that there are racial-cultural differences not only between verbal languages, but also in how non-verbal methods communicate. This is obviously most relevant to disciplines working with minority ethnic groups, of any age, but perhaps especially with older people who are less likely to have learnt new behaviours. Examples of how communication may break down for this reason include the difference between the head-shake in most Western countries which means 'no', and its use in some Asian countries to mean 'yes'. Similarly the use of the thumbs-up sign to convey pleasure would be frowned upon in Bangladesh where it is an insult!

If verbal communication is not possible it may be replaced by a formal non-verbal system or language, such as Makaton (which is often used with mentally handicapped people) or deaf sign language. However the ability to use such languages effectively will depend again on sensory reception (usually visual or tactile), cortical functions and motor output.

AGEING AND COMMUNICATION

The way in which people communicate develops and changes with age. The effect of age on all aspects of the communication chain already discussed, can be seen in 'normal' older people — that is, in the absence of any pathology. It is interesting to observe experienced professional carers of elderly people, who tend subconsciously to adapt their communication to the other's needs. The ways in which carers can adapt become more obvious when the reasons for such an approach are made clear. For this reason the effect of ageing on the communication chain will be described.

Sensory-perceptual changes

All the special senses — vision, hearing, touch, olfaction and taste — appear to become less sensitive as people age. This seems true, despite the influence of response caution, which is more marked in elderly subjects.

Hearing and vision will most obviously affect communication. There are regular alterations in the structures of the ear and eye. In the case of hearing these changes contribute to a decreased ability to hear higher frequency sounds — a condition known as presbyacusis, which is common in older people. The quality of the auditory signal becomes more crucial, as aged people appear to be less able to cope with distorted signals or distracted stimuli. The ways in which one can adapt to improve communication in relation to hearing loss will be discussed more fully later in this chapter, but it is basic to check that hearing aids are worn correctly, are working and can be operated by the wearer or a reliable carer.

Visual changes also occur, and there is an increasing risk of ocular disease (such as glaucoma or cataract). The ability to use non-verbal clues may be reduced, which is particularly important if there is also an auditory deficit. Again older people are less able to cope with poor quality input, so lighting will become more crucial, as will the correct prescription of glasses.

Perception may be defined as the way in which the central nervous system makes use of incoming sensory information. The ability to integrate input from various sources, and make processing decisions, is affected by age changes in the central nervous system, by response rigidity and by a reduced ability to alter initial perceptions (perhaps because of less efficient sensory feedback). The effect of this on communication is that older people should not be asked to cope with too much sensory information at once, or with conflicting input which may be used deliberately, for example, in sarcasm.

Comprehension

It would seem likely that the ability to comprehend language will be affected by changes in the central nervous system, and in cognitive functions. Cohen (1979), for instance, lists speech discrimination, response time, attention, memory, distractibility, and redundancy as factors in comprehension. While there appears to be little change in the knowledge of word meanings, there is increased likelihood of error in understanding unusual or complex grammatical or semantic structures. Cohen (1979) and others have suggested that older people require more explicitly stated information, and are less able to draw inferences. Providing additional, supporting ('redundant') information and context does appear to facilitate comprehension (Cohen and Faulkner 1983).

As it is harder to respond to new stimuli it is crucial that older people are allowed more time — both in general to adapt to a situation, and specifically to take in and understand language. It will also help to avoid more complex ways of phrasing information; and speaking clearly, and perhaps somewhat more slowly, will reduce the likelihood of misunderstanding. It is worth pointing out a truism, however, often ignored by people talking to elderly individuals, which is that age *per se* does not stop a person taking an interest in all aspects of life, and wanting to discuss often complicated matters. The tendency so often seen is for carers to 'talk down' to older people, and this should be avoided at all costs.

While able to understand adequately, unless there is an additional pathology, there may occasionally be a communication failure which is due to what might be described as 'the generation gap' — that is, when people use slang vocabulary, for example, the elderly person may use the slang of their generation!

Cognition

The impact of cognitive changes on language comprehension has been mentioned, but cognition is also bound up in the ability to use language expressively.

Memory, for example, will affect communication directly in its links with the ability to store and recall language units (verbal or non-verbal); and indirectly in determining whether a person appropriately takes account of shared background knowledge in a conversation (failure to do this can lead to excessive repetition, or to unexplained utterances). There appear to be age-related changes in response time, scanning of stored information, and more specifically in recall from episodic memory, acquisition of new information, and the organisation of semantic memory (Davis 1984). Unfortunately, there has been very little research into the effect of age on attention — which anecdotal evidence suggests is reduced. If this is found to be so it may have implications for questions such as how long to expect older people to follow a conversation.

While many clinicians seem to feel that older people are less good at problem-solving (perhaps because of less efficient verbal reasoning skills, among other factors), Williams, Denney and Schadler (1983) found that their elderly subjects felt they were more capable of problem-solving than when younger. It may be that cognitive changes reflect a more functional approach, enabling people to cope with actual daily life and problems more efficiently, but maintaining fewer redundant skills.

Expressive language

Although the knowledge or ability to recognise words is quite consistent, there may be a decline in the variety of words used spontaneously. There is also some evidence that older people experience more difficulty finding the word they want, and are more likely to substitute words — such as using 'boy' instead of 'girl' (Walker 1984). There is

47

also a tendency to use more words when fewer would allow effective transmission of a message (Obler and Albert 1981).

Sentence structure is more likely to show incomplete grammatical constructions; however, age-related changes in this — or word use — are not sufficient to impair communication to the extent that a breakdown occurs.

Motor output

Central mechanisms (such as arousal level), psychological (e.g. response caution) and physiological ageing may all contribute to an increased reaction time. Physical disorders and complaints are common in older people, and often affect movement range, speed and precision.

Speech is affected by respiratory (there is decreased elasticity and power which, together with joint and muscle changes, reduces pulmonary function), and by phonatory and articulatory mechanism changes. The effects of such differences are probably compounded by less efficient sensory feedback mechanisms, which are needed to amend and refine vocal tract gestures.

The parameters of speech most affected by age (Ryan and Burk 1974) are slowed rate, voice tremor, laryngeal tension, air loss and imprecise articulation of consonants. Pitch range is reduced — more markedly in men than in women (Greene 1982). Any discussion of the speech of elderly people would be incomplete without mention of the effect of ill-fitting or absent false teeth — but the remedy is equally obvious!

Psychosocial

Throughout life people enter a sequence of social roles, certain patterns tending to reflect stages of development, with major cultural and socio-economic differences. Age tends to bring a significant diminution in social activity (Dolen and Beavison 1982). There is a need for more study of pragmatics — that is, how language is used in relation to the social context — in relation to how elderly people communicate. Often, professionals involved in the care of elderly people seem to ignore conventions of conversation which are automatic when talking to friends. Older people, whether in hospital, residential care or at home, have the right to choose whether to participate in an interaction, the direction of that conversation, and the subject matter. It is important, for example, that older people who express views on death should be allowed to do so in an accepting atmosphere, and not be ignored or 'jollied' out of it.

It is important to recognise that the ageing process *per se* does not result 'in a defective ability to communicate, but in a different system' (Gravell 1988). Nor is ageing a homogeneous process — each individual will age in different ways. However it is largely accepted that there are these changes in communication, which will then, of course, underlay any alterations due to a specific communication disorder.

DISORDERS OF COMMUNICATION

The disorders of communication with which disciplines working with elderly people are most likely to have contact are listed in Table 3.1. Any individual diagnosed as having one or more of these disorders will present somewhat differently, and thus it is important to stress at this point that the following discussion will be, of necessity, very general. Each person should be assessed whenever possible by the speech therapist who can then offer more specific advice and management plans. (The way in which speech therapists may approach working with older patients will be addressed later in this chapter.)

The disorders will be briefly defined and described, and ways in which carers can adapt to maximise communication potential will be outlined. Communication is a two-way process, and may be improved by adapting the behaviour of the handicapped person and/or the carer.

Hearing loss

Presbyacusis, which was defined earlier as the reduction in the ability to hear sounds of higher frequency, is common among elderly people. It results in a distorted version of speech being heard (without high frequency sounds such as 's', 'z', 'sh').

In general, sensorineural hearing losses are more common than conductive losses — the former due to inner ear changes or disease,

Table 3.1: Disorders of communication

Communication level	Corresponding disorder	Common causes in elderly people
Sensory Input	Hearing Loss	Presbyacusis Occupation Related
	Visual Impairment	Glaucoma Cataract
Comprehension	Dysphasia (Aphasia)	CVA Trauma Tumour Infection
(Cognition)	(Dementia)	(Multi-Infarct) (Alzheimer's)
Expression		
Voluntary Motor Programming	Articulatory Dyspraxia (Apraxia)	CVA
Motor Output	Dysarthria (Anarthria)	CVA Respiratory Disease Ca. Larynx
	Dysphonia (Aphonia)	Parkinson's Disease Iatrogenic
Opportunity and Motivation		Depression Institutionalisation Isolation

and the latter to middle ear. A not infrequent accompanying problem is tinnitus. It is worth noting that various drugs prescribed for older people may cause ototoxicity (for example, some loop diuretics, and antibiotics).

Hearing loss can have a profound effect on pyschosocial adjustment. Often there is a long gap before help is sought (Vernon *et al.* 1981) which further delays the development of coping strategies. In terms of communication the effect on the listener role is obvious, but there is also evidence that hearing loss affects speech, as a result of inability to make use of sensory feedback to maintain standards of clarity and intelligibility. Furthermore, non-verbal communication may be adversely affected — for example in the loss of eye contact if the person is concentrating on lip-reading efforts.

Rehabilitation should include audiological assessment, and

appropriate provision of amplification aids; counselling and instruction in aid use; and education about making use of compensatory techniques, such as lip-reading, awareness of non-verbal communication, auditory training and speech conservation. Environmental aids, such as telephone attachments or flashing light door bells, may be useful.

Talking to the hearing impaired There are numerous ways by which communication with a hearing-impaired person, of any age, can be made easier. The surroundings should be made as quiet as possible, with minimal background noise — this is obviously difficult to achieve in institutions, but can be helped, for example, by switching off televisions which are not being watched. Before speaking the person's attention should be gained, by touch for instance, and it will help to be face to face, rather than standing over a person. Light should be on your face to allow lip-reading, and clear sight of facial expression and gesture. Speakers who cover their mouth or are chewing are almost impossible to follow.

A common error is for people to shout, which further distorts the speech sounds. It is much better to speak at a good level, clearly and slowly, and without over-exaggerated mouth movements. If one ear is better (which is usual) speak to that side. Long, involved sentences should be avoided; and if a message does not get through it is often best to rephrase it in shorter utterances. Gestures and signs can be useful throughout a conversation, as of course can writing messages.

Hearing loss is much harder to cope with in group settings, and care should be taken to make sure the hearing-impaired person is clued in. Sudden subject changes often lead to confusing misunderstandings.

Finally, it is worth remembering that many people try to cover up their hearing loss, and need sympathetic handling. There is still stigma attached to the stereotype of being 'old and deaf'.

It is important to point out that hearing aids do not replace lost hearing. Indeed amplification distorts sound, and is not selective, so that background noise may be particularly distressing. Thus aid wearers will still benefit from speakers taking the steps described above. Aids need regular maintenance, and it should not be assumed that because an aid is worn, it is working!

Visual impairment

'Ocular disease increases more or less exponentially with age, and thus the very old are at a very considerable risk of one or more' (Williamson and Caird 1986). The relevance of this, and of age-related changes in visual acuity, accommodation, contrast sensitivity and adaptation, to communication, is most obviously in relation to the written word. Thus reading or writing become difficult or impossible. However, there may also be considerable impact on a person's ability to make use of non-verbal clues. Visual impairment may mean such clues are misinterpreted and thus lead to misunderstandings or effectively block reception of a message.

Visual handicap, if there is also a hearing loss, will be particularly handicapping. As in the case of hearing loss, rehabilitation will involve support in making use of what residual visual ability remains, and education in using other sensory channels to compensate (e.g. touch, as in the use of Braille).

When talking to visually handicapped people — be they old or young — it is important to ensure good lighting free from glare, and to use touch. If hearing is intact it is important to remember, when talking to the person, that they will need to have more information supplied — they will not, for example, follow gesture, or be able to appreciate fully any comment based on your immediate observation of events.

Aphasia

Aphasia or dysphasia (the terms denote severity, but tend to be used interchangeably) refers to a disruption of language as a result of brain damage. The most common cause is cerebrovascular accident, and thus it is more likely that older people will present with aphasia. Perhaps the clearest way to describe the impairment is by first defining 'language'.

Language is a code chosen to represent and communicate ideas and feelings, which is accepted and agreed upon by all users to enable them to understand and to structure messages. It does not refer to the actual physical execution of that code — thus any disruption of articulation or of handwriting is not due to the aphasia (they may of course share initial aetiology). The fact that language *per se* is disrupted in aphasia means that comprehension and use of both spoken and written forms will be impaired. The particular symptoms (e.g. comprehension may be relatively less impaired than the ability to structure expressive language or vice versa) and the severity will depend on the site and extent of the cortical lesion.

The manifestations of aphasia can be bizarre and difficult to understand. While numerous ways of categorising different syndrome complexes exist, and recognising that pure forms are rarely found, it may be useful to consider 'receptive' and 'expressive' aphasia, which are terms commonly used in medical circles. It is quite extraordinary to see a patient, however, who does not have some difficulty in both areas.

Receptive aphasia Damage to Wernicke's area is thought to be the root of receptive comprehension difficulty. The incoming signal is heard, but there is a failure to attach meaning to what is heard. People with this form of aphasia will often be able to make use of non-verbal clues, and may pick up the gist of conversation. However, it will rarely help to write down messages, as all verbal language is affected.

There will be evidence of the comprehension loss in expressive language, and often there is a lack of insight into errors. Inappropriate words (linked in meaning or sound to the intended word) or neologisms (newly coined non-words) may be used, and in extreme cases output may take the form of extended neologistic jargon. This is often accompanied by facial expression and intonation patterns which are appropriate to what the person intended (and believes he is) saying.

Expressive aphasia In the presence of relatively preserved ability to understand language, there may be a disorder of the ability to structure expressive language. This is linked to damage to Broca's area. Insight tends to be better retained and output is often hesitant and non-fluent (unlike the fluency of Wernicke's or receptive aphasics). Word-finding difficulty is common, when patients feel they know the word but cannot actually produce it. Grammatically, utterances are incomplete or misconstructed. At a severe level people may be restricted to a few stereotyped, perseverative utterances.

Talking to the aphasic patient As both comprehension and expression are usually impaired to a greater or lesser degree, it is important first for the speaker to adapt their output to enable the aphasic person to understand as much as possible. This is relevant for every health or social service professional, instructing or discussion rehabilitation and future management with the patient.

Quiet, non-distracting surroundings will help, and the person's attention must be gained before attempting communication. Speech should be somewhat slower, and utterances short, simple (but not childish) and direct. Positive phrasing ('Do this') is better than making more negative, complex requests. More repetition may be needed, but of the meaning (that is, by rephrasing) rather than of specific words. Direct questions (yes/no, or giving a forced, limited choice) are often most useful. Vague, abstract subjects will be much harder for the aphasic person to follow.

Gestures, facial expression and other non-verbal methods should be used whenever appropriate to reinforce the spoken word. In hospital there is a very definite routine, and this may serve to help an aphasic to understand what is required of him and her — it can also effectively disguise comprehension loss, and staff must be aware that this is a possibility.

Expressively, it is important to encourage all attempts at communication, whether by word, intonation, gesture or facial expression. It is also important not to guess too readily what the person intends to say — if their utterance is unclear questions phrased to require only a yes/no response can be used to clarify their meaning.

It is not uncommon for aphasic patients to swear more than they used to — often this is an automatic, stereotyped response and may upset the patient, as well as others who may not understand why this happens.

It is also important to realise that people with aphasia fluctuate considerably — the ability to say a word one day does *not* mean that word has been relearnt and will always be accessible.

Encouragement is crucial, for patients with aphasia face an isolating and terrifying world. The speech therapist's assessment should more specifically indicate ways in which individuals may be best approached. As was said earlier, communication is a two-way process, and even if impaired people cannot alter their communication behaviour, the other person may restore the balance by adapting his or her own.

Dementia

Dementia is a 'chronic, progressive brain disease, characterised by intellectual deterioration, impaired memory, and disorientation' (Pitt 1982). To this list could be added communication failure (Bayles *et al.* 1982). In the past this was often described as aphasia, but it is qualitatively different, despite the fact that there may be shared features.

There are various conditions which fall into the category of dementia, the most common of which are Alzheimer's disease — which accounts for approximately half of all dementia cases (Bayles *et al.* 1982) — and Multi-Infarct (MID), which can result from a series of cerebrovascular accidents or transient ischaemic attacks.

As communicative and other symptoms will depend on the location of any brain damage, it is almost impossible to specify the nature of breakdown. However, in general terms it can be said that communication in dementia is characterised by disruption first of pragmatic and semantic aspects, and only in the late stage by phonological or grammatical errors. An early word-finding difficulty (anomia) may be apparent, alongside a general vagueness and rambling. More complex linguistic forms — such as analogy or sarcasm — will be harder to follow. In the later stages of dementia patients will be insensitive to the communicative context, unable to follow verbal language, and may be mute or use repetitive jargon. Rarely, language disorder may be the initial sign of the onset of dementia; and there are cases in which a progressive aphasia has been found to persist for years prior to any evidence of a deterioration in generalised intellectual ability.

Talking to dementing patients When communicating with dementia sufferers it is important to minimise distractions and gain their attention. Concrete and familiar terms and topics — avoiding abrupt changes in subject matter — will be easier. Talking about the 'old days' may be the most successful subject, and thus provide them with a positive enjoyable communicative experience.

Frequent reminders of time, place and person will be necessary; and the establishment of a simple, consistent routine is crucial.

Perhaps of all the causes of communication difficulty dementia is the most difficult for both lay and professional carers to adapt to, and thus carers will need a lot of support and encouragement. Explanations and advice from a speech therapist can help to ensure communication breakdown is understood, and carers can then be taught how to modify their own communication skills more specifically.

A more detailed description of the language of dementia, and of the speech therapist's role, may be found in Gravell (1988).

Articulatory dyspraxia

Articulatory dyspraxia is rather a controversial concept, but may be defined as 'an articulatory disorder resulting from impairment, as a result of brain damage, of the capacity to program the positioning of speech musculature and the sequencing of muscle movements for the volitional production of phonemes. No significant weakness, slowness of incoordination in reflex and automatic acts' (Darley 1969).

In practice, assessment and diagnosis are complicated by the frequent co-occurrence of dysphasia, and it is likely there will be both comprehension and expressive language disorders as well as an articulatory dyspraxia (although not inevitable). Thus the same general advice will apply in talking to these patients as to 'pure' aphasics.

In the rare event of a pure articulatory dyspraxia it may be possible to use the written word, unlike with aphasics.

Dysarthria/dysphonia

While aphasia is a language disorder, dysarthria is purely a disorder of speech — that is of the actual physical production of the sounds chosen as symbols for a particular verbal language.

The dysarthrias are a group of related motor-speech disorders, which are due to a disturbance of muscular control necessary for the production of intelligible speech. A wide variety of neuropathologies can cause dysarthria, and elderly people face an increased risk of suffering certain of these conditions, perhaps most notably CVA and Parkinson's disease. The normal age changes in speech have been described by some as resulting in 'minimal dysarthria', although it seems strange to describe a normal developmental change as a disorder, particularly as age *per se* does not lead to lack of functional intelligibility.

Various different symptom complexes may occur — Parkinson's disease, for example, tends to present with breathiness, monotony, altered rate (often festinance), initiation difficulty and imprecise articulation. If a CVA leads to dysarthric symptoms they are attributable to unilateral or bilateral facial weakness, which results in slurred, slowed articulation. As dysarthria is an output disorder, however, the ability to understand, and to make use of the written word (either reading or writing) is not impaired — unless there are other co-occurring reasons, such as confusion, hemiplegia or ataxia.

Dysphonia is also purely an output disorder, and describes a disorder of voice production. (Aphonia is total loss of voice.) There is often a dysphonia alongside dysarthria after a CVA or in other neurological conditions. Older patients are also more likely to present with dysphonia due to laryngeal carcinoma, which may be treated by radio-therapy and/or surgery. Again, understanding, and use of the written word are not affected.

Talking to dysarthrics Perhaps most important, because it is a trap so often fallen into, is that listeners should not pretend to understand when they do not. This is usually obvious to the speaker, and may cause great frustration. Comprehension is intact, so no specific precautions need be taken when talking to a dysarthric person.

It will be important that the dysarthric is given time as their speech will often be slow and laboured. A quiet background will help, and the listener may be helped if able to watch facial movements. If a message is not understood various techniques may be tried. If any of the utterance was intelligible it is worth repeating, so the speaker is aware how much you have understood, and need not tire himself by repeating unnecessary information. Questioning may be a way of clarifying a message. If necessary the speaker should be asked to slow down, even to the extent of saying one word at a time, or spelling out a word.

If a person is physically able to write, this medium may be used as an adjunct to speech efforts, or in some instances instead of speech. For those who cannot write because of physical handicap there are increasing numbers of mechanical and electronic communication aids. No study has been done on whether such aids are less acceptable to elderly people, or harder to learn to use because of the evidence of less efficient learning skills.

It is worth mentioning the higher rates of illiteracy among elderly people, mainly due to less educational opportunity earlier this century, and this should be borne in mind in relation to rehabiliation work, or great embarrassment and distress may be caused.

Lack of opportunity/motivation to communicate

While lack of opportunity does not cause a specific communication disorder, it may serve as just as effective a barrier to communication. Elderly people face a greater risk because more live alone — which leads to isolation — but also because there is an increased likelihood that they will be institutionalised. Institutional life often removes the need to communicate, by providing an ultra-supportive environment that requires residents/patients to make no decisions or choices. Often residents feel they have no opportunity to communicate because there are no suitable communication partners (Lubinski *et al.* 1981).

Lack of motivation to communicate may stem from depression, experience of failure (if, for example, there is a specific disorder such as aphasia or dysarthria) or be due to the effects of a restricted lifestyle, in which lack of stimulation means there is little about which to communicate.

Those who work with older people, particularly those in institutions, can help provide both opportunity and experience of successful and enjoyable communication. As much choice as is possible for each individual should be allowed, to encourage the need to interact, and alterations in daily routine can provide subject matter, as can such activities as reminiscence therapy which encourages discussion by making use of an individual's memories.

Working with elderly people with communication disorders

Some general advice on talking to older people, and specifically to people suffering from certain communication disorders, has been offered. All disciplines involved in the care of elderly people must be aware of the importance of communication, and understand how to approach individuals with such disorders. It is evident that different disorders require different approaches, but so do different individuals.

Factors such as personality, co-occurring illnesses or handicaps, cultural-racial background, and the available support from family and friends, will be important in determining how older (or younger) people react to their disorder. Professionals working with them must be aware how all-enveloping is a loss of communication, in order to appreciate the change in lifestyle it brings. Psychological and social reactions are common, and must be sensitively handled.

This chapter will close by briefly describing the way in which the speech therapist works with older patients, and how he or she must work within the multidisciplinary team in order to provide the best possible care for each individual patient.

SPEECH THERAPY WITH ELDERLY PEOPLE

In the United Kingdom most speech therapists who work with older people are hospital-based, seeing a mixture of in-patients and out-patients. Often, bringing aged and frail patients in to a hospital clinic is counter-productive, and there has been some increase in domiciliary visiting, which has many advantages for this client group (Stevens 1985; Gravell 1988).

In addition to traditional therapy — that is, direct one-to-one or group work with the patient — there has been a growing awareness of the need for what might be described as indirect therapeutic involvement. Figure 3.3 outlines the main management decisions with which the speech therapist will be faced.

Assessment may take the form of informal observation, or of standardised testing of language, speech, voice, and — increasingly — of functional communication (overall ability to communicate in everyday life). Interpretation of tests used with elderly people is not always easy, as very few offer norms for older age groups despite the fact that changes in communicative ability are recognised. Similarly, the materials and equipment used may not be suitable if they fail to take account of visual and other changes.

Direct therapy will be planned specifically for the patient, in order to maximise residual abilities. However, for a number of reasons direct therapy is not always appropriate — particularly in the case of elderly people who are more likely to have additional pathologies and handicaps. Speech therapy is an active process, which requires the patient thus to be co-operative and motivated, which links in to insight. Although in some cases it may be seen as re-learning, it is making conscious previously automatic processes which means learning efficiency, attention, memory and cognition

Figure 3.3: The main management decisions facing the speech therapist

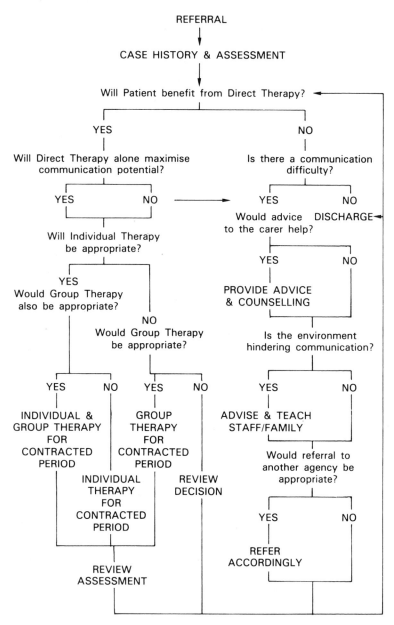

will be important. Certain disorders may make intervention difficult — for example if sensory losses, such as deafness, are unmanaged (by amplification or education), or because of some somatic, and mental, illnesses which reduce motivation or lessen the physical ability to cope with often tiring drills and programmes.

Finally, environmental factors may occasionally preclude direct work — weekly therapy that can not be backed up by family, friends or volunteers may have few benefits, for instance.

The existence of any one of these factors does not necessarily mean therapy is inappropriate. Each person must be considered in relation to their individual situation. However, if there is no benefit to be gained from direct work, then this decision must be firmly taken and fully explained, both to the family and other team members. The communication difficulty remains, and exclusion of one-to-one work does not mean the speech therapist can no longer play a role in the multidisciplinary team's management of that person.

Indirect therapy may take the form of advice and training of the carer(s) in relation to the specific communication difficulty, or in relation to how the environment can be altered to maximise interaction (such things as lighting, background noise, furniture placement and so on). Counselling may help the carer(s) to adjust to the elderly person's residual deficits in a more realistic way. Obviously there may also be the need for referral to other agencies, such as audiologists, or psychologists.

It cannot be stressed too greatly that the *team* approach to management should be adopted whenever possible. Communication is, perhaps, the one aspect of a patient's ability that will affect every possible approach to rehabilitation and continuing care. Whether communication is limited to the most basic level of eye contact, or involves more complex use of language, all members of the team must be aware of the person's abilities and needs.

Obviously the team approach is based on the sharing of information and expertise. The speech therapist working with older patients may need to adapt his or her approach as a result of the findings of other team members. The team approach should thus ensure comprehensive care, to allow maximal functional ability in each patient.

SUMMARY

This chapter has focused on the communication of older people, and the most commonly-found disorders of communication in the elderly population. Everyone, regardless of age, needs communication in order to achieve some quality of life. Weiss (1971) discussed the communicative needs of aged people and nicely summarised the role of intervention as 'not so much adding years to their life, but adding life to their years'. This should be the aim of all disciplines, not just the speech therapist, as they adjust and adapt to the different communication patterns of elderly people and of those who are communicatively handicapped.

REFERENCES

Bayles, K.A., Tomoeda, C.K. and Caffrey, J.T. (1982) Language and Dementia Producing Diseases. *Communication Disorders, 7*, (10), 131–46

Cohen, G. (1979) Language Comprehension in Old Age. *Cognitive Psychology, 11*, 412–29

Cohen, G. and Faulkner, D. (1983) Word Recognition: Age Differences in Contextual Facilitation Effects. *British Journal of Psychology, 74*, 239–51

Darley, F.L. (1969) Aphasia Input and Output Disturbances in Speech and Language Processing. Paper to American Speech and Hearing Association, Chicago

Davis, G.A. (1984) Effects of Aging on Normal Language. In A. Holland (ed.), *Language Disorders in Adults*. College Hill Press, 79–112

Dolen, L.S. and Beavison, D.J. (1982) Social Interaction and Social Cognition in Aging: A Contextual Analysis. *Human Development, 25*, 430–42

Gravell, R.E. (1988) *Communication Problems in Elderly People — Practical Approaches to Management*. Croom Helm, London

Greene, M.C.L. (1982) Aging of the Voice — A Review. In M. Edwards (ed.), *Communication Changes in Elderly People*. College of Speech Therapy, Monograph, 62–8

Lubinski, R. (1978/9) Why So Little Interest in Whether or Not Old People Talk? *International Journal of Aging and Human Development, 9*, (3), 237–44

Lubinski, R. (1981) Language and Aging: An Environment Approach to Intervention. *Topics in Language Disorders*, Aspens Systems Corporation, 89–97

Lubinski, R., Morrison, E.B. and Rigrodsky, S. (1981) Perception of Spoken Communication by Elderly Chronically Ill Patients in an Institutional Setting. *Journal of Speech and Hearing Disorders, 46*, November, 405–12

Obler, L.K. and Albert, M.L. (1981) Language and Aging: A Neurobehavioural Analysis. In D.S. Beasley and G.A. Davis (eds.), *Aging: Communication Processes and Disorders*. Grune & Stratton Inc., 107–22

Pitt, B. (1982) *Psychogeriatrics*, 2nd edition, Churchill Livingstone, Edinburgh

Ryan, W.J. and Burk, K.W. (1974) Perception and Acoustic Correlates of Aging. *Journal of Communicative Disorders, 7*, 181

Stevens, S. (1985) A Domiciliary Service for the Elderly. *CST Bulletin, 41*, (September)

Vernon, M., Griffin, D.H. and Yoken, C. (1981) Hearing Loss. *Journal of Family Practice, 12*, (6), 1152–8

Walker, S.A. (1984) The Communicative Status of Older People: Differentiation and Rehabilitation. *International Rehabilitation and Medicine, 6*, 139–43

Weiss, A.E. (1971) Communication Needs of the Geriatric Population. *Journal of American Geriatric Society, 19*, 640–5

Williams, S.A., Denney, N.W. and Schadler, M. (1983) Elderly Adults' Perception of Their Own Cognitive Development During the Adult Years. *International Journal of Aging and Human Development, 16*, (2), 147–58

Williamson, J. and Caird, F.I. (1986) Epidemiology of Ocular Diseases in Old Age. In F.I. Caird and J. Williamson, *The Eye and Its Disorders in the Elderly*. Wright, Bristol, 1–8

4

Assessment of the Older Patient

Amanda Squires and Madeline Taylor

Assessment can be defined as a systematic gathering and interpretation of data (Rogers 1980) and skilled team members can contribute to this in their own area of expertise.

Geriatric medicine was conceived by Dr Marjory Warren on the basis of assessment and rehabilitation, and the purpose of assessment has been described by Rubenstein (1983) as to provide a diagnosis, plan for therapy and services, consider appropriate placement and provide a baseline against which change can be monitored. From the findings of the assessment, aims and objectives can be set and realistic treatment plans devised. In the UK there has never been a policy of encouraging elderly people to enter long-term care (Murphy, 1986) and although management of elderly people in the community is the ideal many patients will be admitted to hospital on a geriatric or medical ward and therefore the hospital assessment procedure will be described here. (The community-based approach is described more fully in Chapters 11, 12 and 13.)

Hospitalisation can encourage dependence, therefore early assessment, and intervention if appropriate, are essential deterrents. Initially it is important to gain information from the referring agent with as many details as possible about the patient's history, reason for admission and consequent referral to relevant departments. Quinn *et al.* (1979) recommended that the actual reason for referral, by whom and why at that particular time are recorded. There must be consultation with other staff, the patient's medical notes, the family or other significant carer, and the patient, to gain a full picture of the patient's abilities, problems, lifestyle and expectations and also those of the carers.

The admission may have been caused by a gradual breakdown in the home situation which causes an initial decrease in ability until a point is reached where personal care fails to be maintained. Alternatively, admission may have been caused by a crisis breakdown — more usually caused by sudden illness in the old person — but may also be due to problems with the helpers, the environment or a lapse in communication between the agencies. In the latter case 'Home Help on holiday' is a typical but unnecessary cause of admission, and intervention should be speedy and appropriate to the cause. Lay people see three main problems in looking after an old person at home — mental confusion, immobility and falls — and the addition of incontinence may precipitate the referral (Millard 1982).

When the situation at home does break down it is vitally important to refer the patient immediately to prevent deterioration of his condition. It may well be that fast referral can allow community agencies to intervene and prevent admission being necessary, but where admission is needed referral to physiotherapy and occupational therapy should occur without delay if the medical condition allows, so that a realistic assessment of capabilities can be undertaken and a programme of activities commenced immediately with full team involvement.

The state of the patient prior to the incident which caused the referral/admission is also essential for planning, and Hodkinson and Hodkinson (1980) found that a high level of activity, low age, no wait for admission, high mental state, and admission from home all supported better prospects for discharge. It is also known that while waiting for admission domestic skills deteriorate (Challis 1981) and it may be difficult to re-establish them.

Prior to the formal assessment it is important to develop a good rapport with the patient. Team members must liaise with each other to determine which areas each will cover depending on available expertise and resources. There will inevitably be areas of overlap between professionals, and focusing on the patient rather than on inter-professional jealousies will prevent barriers being created. Discussion on assessment findings between team members is essential.

The level of communication possible between assessor and patient must be determined from the outset. The attitude of both to each other will often determine the future relationship and sight, hearing, speech, language, and mental status must also be identified. Aids to communication such as teeth, hearing aids and glasses should be available and in good working order. It is worth noting that Beswick (1987) found that nine-tenths of elderly people did not use their hearing aids regularly one year after fitting, but he also felt that with care most elderly people with hearing problems could be helped. Aids necessary for the patient to function as independently as possible should also be available and while relatives are collecting communication aids it is prudent to request other aids such as clothes, shoes, walking aids, calipers and wheelchairs to save further journeys. All such aids and appliances should be checked and sent for repair early in the admission if they are going to be needed so that delay in discharge is not caused by poor management.

Patients with poor communication present a particularly difficult problem to the assessor and help from the speech therapist and/or psychologist should be urgently sought. It may be found beneficial to use other forms of communication such as sign language, writing, gesture or physical contact to aid communication.

The venue for the assessment is also important. A busy, noisy ward is not conducive to discussing personal matters, and access to a quiet but informal room with no interruptions from bleeps and telephones is ideal, but medical and environmental considerations may preclude this option. Wherever the interview takes place introducing oneself and the job one does is essential. Asking the patient about himself and how he sees his admission and referral will be most revealing. It should be remembered that people of the age under consideration have vivid recollections of the death sentence prescribed when admission to a geriatric ward or hospital occurred, and may have low expectations of the help that can be offered. Many geriatric hospitals in the United Kingdom are housed in former 'workhouses' and have similar connotations (Squires 1986b). The patient should be encouraged to express why he felt he was admitted, what problems exist at home and the support systems he had had, if any. He should also be asked how he thinks the problem could be solved — many patients have sat and pondered at length and have original and workable solutions — if only we asked them.

When all the information has been obtained by team members it should be shared so that an ultimate aim with short-term and long-term goals can be determined, and tasks allocated. The aids, adaptations and community support needed should also be considered early so that delay in discharge is not caused by another consequence of poor management.

HOW TO ASSESS

The assessment is carried out by observation and examination of the patient in a variety of different situations. The patient must be included, not excluded, in this assessment by being asked questions on his ability at home in various activities. The family and significant carers should also be included at this stage, but it should be noted that Rubenstein (*et al.* 1984) found that the patient had the highest opinion of his abilities, and the relatives the lowest. Rubenstein felt that the patient's attitude could be due to optimism, shifted time-frame or concealment, and the relatives' view was due to being overburdened.

As the patient may initially be admitted to hospital the assessment will have to be carried out there, but prior to discharge assessments at home are essential for a realistic view. Facilities in hospital should be as similar to those at home as possible such as the kitchen, bathroom, bedroom, toilet and distance to it, bed, chair and any necessary aids. Hall (1976) and others have identified three main areas for assessment and these are:

(i) Social functioning.
(ii) Mental functioning.
(iii) Physical functioning.

SOCIAL FUNCTIONING

The social needs of the older patient must be taken into account when assessing them. These needs are discussed under the following headings.

Individuality

Each patient must be treated as an individual and the patient's ideas and wishes taken into consideration. It may not be necessary to assess all areas of physical and mental functioning; it will depend on the diagnosis, signs and symptoms the patient displays. The patient's personality must also be considered. It is unwise to assume that the patient knows who the assessor is or what the assessor's job entails — each assessor should state his name, explain his role and why he is there. Surnames should always be used initially, with the correct prefix. (A lot of ground will be lost by imposing marital status on a spinster!) The patient may ask you to call him by his first name or nickname, which should be accepted as a gesture of friendliness, and it will be the decision of the individual staff member in that individual situation whether to reciprocate.

Physical contact

With the older patient, physical contact is important. By putting your arm around him or holding his hand confidence and comfort can be gained by the patient. Health-care staff are amongst the few who are 'permitted' to touch their clients, and this powerful tool should be used within reason.

Body language

Staff should always talk to the patient at eye level (i.e. sitting if the patient is sitting, and facing him directly at a distance comfortable to both). Speak in a clear voice and give concise instructions. There should be no need to shout, although some people habitually shout at all old people assuming they have a hearing difficulty. Try to approach in a friendly manner to put the patient at ease. Never approach from behind as this can frighten and can cause vestibular disturbance and falls if the patient's neck is turned quickly.

Dignity and self-respect

Always be respectful to the older person and do not try to rush him. Remember to pull the curtains around the bed if an intimate examination or procedure is to take place. Remember the whole ward will be watching. Never assume that you are the only assessor — the other patients and the one being assessed are summing the assessor up at the same time! When encouraging the patient to carry out an activity, do it with dignity and allow the patient plenty of time. However busy staff are, the patient is the most important person at that time and he should have the undivided attention of that person, not at all easy to implement in today's rushed pace of life. It must never be forgotten that it is the patient who is our reason for professional existence.

Failure

It is important to remember that the older patient may frequently fail to achieve the tasks staff take for granted. It is important to always try and encourage activities within the patient's capabilities and provide constant positive feedback during the task, when the task is complete or when it is obvious that the patient has tried very hard. This will boost morale and self-esteem, enabling the patient to go on and achieve more. The patient should always be aware of what the task is and when he has achieved it. It is essential that other members of the team are briefed on what may appear minimal progress but to the patient and relevant staff member may be a huge advance.

Environment

Consideration should be given to the environment for the social well-being of the patient as well as the staff. The ward environment should be as homely as possible. Carpeting makes the ward look inviting, warmer and is quieter. It is possible to buy carpets which can easily be cleaned where spilt water or urine does not sink in, but they do require regular cleaning. As this item has implications for various professional and ancillary disciplines full discussion is essential prior to a decision being made, and regular monitoring of progress.

Small tables and chairs for about four to six people with tablecloths and place-mats as one would have at home make the ward look less institutional. All chairs should be selected by the ward team to reflect the needs of all the patients who might use them. Chairs in the dining area should not be exempt from this plan, nor should visitors' chairs — elderly patients tend to have elderly visitors who may find difficulty managing on plastic stacking chairs. The ideal is a 'pool' of chairs so each patient can be supplied with the best one for his needs, and have it replaced as his abilities change. Relatives needing advice on suitable chairs to purchase can be shown examples in the 'pool'. A new initiative has been developed where a six-weekly chair clinic is held using an assessment chair which can be adjusted for height, width, seat slant, foot and head rests and types of castor. A chair can then be made from the measurements obtained (*Therapy Weekly* 1987). Evaluation of the long-term effects of this procedure will be of great value for the future of chair design for disabled people.

Pictures and mirrors on the wall and flowers brighten up the ward and many schemes such as volunteers and League of Friends of the hospital exist to implement this. If possible the sitting areas should be divided into two or three small sections. This can be done by using bookshelves or room dividers suitably constructed so as not to act as a tripping risk to patients due to protruding supports. One area could be used for the television and playing music, another for quieter pursuits such as reading. There should be a cassette and record player available and plenty of books, including large print, and up-to-date newspapers and magazines. Orientation can be quite disturbed by reading out-of-date news, as some waiting rooms highlight!

There should also be 'talking books' available for the visually handicapped, and those unable to read. Some elderly people like to be alone, and this should be respected; forcing them to socialise may well be counter-productive.

Personalised clothing, or the patient's own clothing, should be available to assist in encouraging independence, dignity and choice. Some hospitals request relatives to take all the patient's own clothing home to avoid complaints of loss or damage in the hospital laundry. Clothing may be supplied from a communal cupboard, in which case sizing is seldom adequate. Sharing personal items like underwear, which would not be tolerated in society generally, should not be inflicted on elderly people in hospital. Personalised clothing bridges the gap between the patient's own clothing and that supplied by the institution. The clothing should be selected by, and labelled for, that patient for the duration of their stay. It is compatible with the laundry system, with any losses being debited to the hospital, not the patient. The Disabled Living Foundation has done much to promote and publicise this initiative (Turnbull 1982).

Where possible, unrestricted visiting should be encouraged, and carers assisting in patient treatment and care should be welcomed — after all they have probably been undertaking it for some time at home, and may have to continue after discharge. If a patient has few or no visitors a befriending scheme could be set up if the patient wishes. This can involve individual volunteers or schoolchildren who come to visit patients and form a relationship with them, and it can follow on after discharge. With such schemes it is important to have a supervisor who can impress on participants the importance of confidentiality and also have explained to them the ward and hospital routine. Volunteers should be seen for supervision, guidance and support regularly, at least twice a week for those working daily, and they should be encouraged to feed back any problems they encounter. Hospital staff should not see volunteers as a threat, but as an important adjunct to formal treatment. The tiring effect of being a hospital patient should not be overlooked, as anxiety, new environment, poor sleep, changes in medication, and the effects of illness and its treatment all can take its toll. Add to this well-meaning visitors who fill all available visiting time, and the patient may well request convalescence at an inaccessible retreat!

Social skills

Social skills are a necessary part of an elderly patient's life to enable him to function in hospital and at home.

Communication is an essential human ability. It is used with families and friends, sales assistants in shops, hospital staff and other patients to name but a few. The elderly patient may have lost his ability to communicate and to use social skills, because of depression or anxiety brought on by his illness or inability to carry out everyday tasks. The patient may require speech therapy if he has had an illness resulting in communication difficulties. The therapist may need to increase the patient's confidence and self-esteem and thus improve social skills. This can be done by practising all Activities of Daily Living (ADL) where the patient has problems or generally boosting morale by encouraging participation in group activities.

A very anxious patient may require relaxation training to overcome fears of communicating with others. If the patient has specific difficulties he may be able to join a social skills training programme as an in-patient or out-patient.

Activities

A regular programme of purposeful activities carried out with the staff is also important to help the patient's social functioning and integration. This can be done both individually and in groups and occupational therapists have much experience and expertise in this area and should be sought for advice (Table 4.1)

A music therapist can assist greatly in this process by running regular sessions. Music therapists are professional trained therapists with music ability who are then trained to use music as a medium to obtain physical, emotional or social response from patients.

Festivals, such as Easter, Harvest and St George's Day, can be

Table 4.1: Individual activities that can be used to stimulate elderly patients

Reality orientation	Using a large board with details of the day, date, etc
Reminiscence	This can be carried out using themes such jobs, family, marriage, pets, both world wars, etc. Pictures from magazines are used as visual aids and talking points
Crosswords	Using a newspaper or a crossword book
Collage	Using pieces of material, magazine pictures and the like as themes such as autumn, Christmas, etc. Cut out images and glue on sheets of card
Painting and drawing	
Current affairs	Reading about and discussing current events, using newspapers and books
Bingo	
Table games	Card games are especially popular with male patients
Dominoes	Play using large pieces or card substitutes
Sewing/knitting/tapestry	Plus any other hobbies patients had in the past
Music	Singing, playing instruments, listening to music — records/cassettes
Cookery	
Looking after plants in the ward	
Flower arranging	
Correspondence	Assisting patients to write letters to relatives, send birthday cards, etc
Making decorations	Christmas decorations, Easter, Valentine and birthday cards
Reading	Poetry. Provide large print books from the librarian
Make-up	Assist patients to put on make-up if they wish. Use a large mirror. Wash and set hair
Quiz	Make a list of questions using local geography, Royal Family, etc.
Identification	Choose for identification pictures of objects and ask patients to describe their uses. (Vary according to intellectual ability of patients.)

celebrated on the ward or in the hospital chapel with outside musicians. Various theatrical groups (see Useful Addresses) can be invited to perform in hospital wards and involve the patients where possible. These events should be enjoyable for staff as well as patients and much will be gained by the participation of all grades and disciplines.

When participating in any activity, patients, like any members of society, should be given choices. It does not help an elderly person to be forced into group activities against his will. Choices about meals are also important, and menus should be completed by the patient where possible. Going out to local familiar places, if the medical condition

Table 4.2: The broad areas of assessment for the patient's mental state. (After Boardman.)

Appearance and behaviour	General appearance and hygiene; co-operation; aggression; appropriate/inappropriate behaviour; attention-seeking behaviour
Activity performance	Motivation; attention/concentration; ability to follow verbal/written instructions; practical ability
Intellectual ability	Awareness of surroundings/self; calculation; judgement; decision-making; hearing ability; comprehension; memory; recognition; ability to read and write
Physical state	Vision; speech; hearing; sensation; co-ordination; fatigue
Perception	Body awareness; visual; spatial; auditory
Cognitive functioning	Attention and concentration; memory and intelligence; reasoning and visuospatial difficulties; recognition and dyspraxia; motor skills; language
Orientation	Time; place; person
Affect	Apathy; depression; anxiety
Interpersonal behaviour	Group interaction; under/over talkative; initiate conversation; confabulation; communication, dysphasia, receptive/expressive; jargon dysphasia; dysarthria

permits, are also helpful for orientation and rebuilding confidence prior to discharge.

MENTAL FUNCTIONING

All members of the team will be assessing the patient's mental state (Table 4.2) as the type of intervention each can provide will depend on the ability of the patient to understand and co-operate. As with previous assessments, team members will need to discuss areas of overlap and decide who will do what, and communicate the results. Teams including a psychologist will be able to add another dimension to the traditional team composition.

Once the problems, if any, have been identified, the team will have to decide, which, if any, should be treated and by whom. It should be remembered that some responses displayed by the patient may be life-long characteristics, and change after seven or eight decades may not only be impossible but also undesirable. Some problem areas may not affect the patient's lifestyle at home and can be disregarded. There are many formal methods of assessing and recording mental ability in old age which are described later (Chapter 5).

PHYSICAL FUNCTIONING

The physical assessment of the elderly patient is vitally important to enable him to function as independently as possible despite any disability. In the younger patient specific degrees of joint-range and muscle-strength measured against weight and frequency are more appropriate for their current and possible lifestyle. As one ages, function becomes more important (Nicholls 1976) and ADL are the criteria for ability to manage at home, and are therefore the criteria for assessment. It has been noted that there are as many ADL forms as there are occupational therapy departments (Nicholls 1976). Although the British Association of Occupational Therapists attempted standardisation, it proved unacceptable to members as each departmental form had been designed to reflect local needs and were judged better than forms foreign to the assessor. The Association of Chartered Physiotherapists, with a special interest in elderly people, has attempted a General Mobility Index (Figure 4.1) consisting of the six items most frequently assessed by members. This is used as an evaluative aid to the assessment form already in use in individual departments, and has had some success in trials to date (Squires *et al.* 1987).

Whatever procedure is followed team communication is essential as each member will have something to contribute and learn. The assessment should cover the patient's needs during the 24-hour day, to include the areas listed in Table 4.3 and should be related to the needs and help available in the patient's preferred environment.

Home visit assessment

Assessment of the home environment and support is an essential part of the assessment process and is more fully described elsewhere in this book. For our purposes in this chapter, Table 4.3 will suffice.

The General Mobility Index (Squires 1986a; Squires *et al.* 1987) can be adapted to provide an assessment, aim and evaluation guide for most activities.

There are many assessment forms and each person will choose that most suitable to their own needs. What they should have in common is to be able to show the patient's ability in the basic functions to permit an independent lifestyle at home during the 24-hour day. The latter fact should be remembered by those whose work

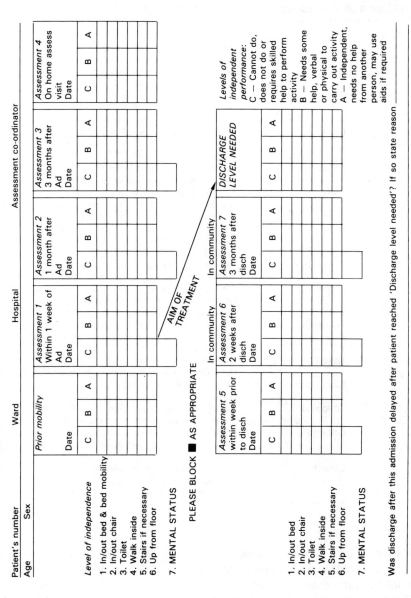

Figure 4.1: General mobility index

Table 4.3: Assessment of the home environment

Mobility	Walking	Ability to walk short distances and the aids, verbal or physical help, needed
	Falls	Ability to look after self, call for help or get up after a fall; and the aids, verbal or physical help, needed
Transfers	Bed	Ability to get in and out of bed and move within it; and the aids (e.g. rope ladder), verbal or physical help, needed
	Chair	Ability to get on and off the chair (at a relevant height); and the aids, verbal or physical help, needed
	Toilet	Ability to get on or off the toilet; and the aids, verbal or physical help, needed
	Bath	Ability to get in or out of the bath; and the aids, verbal or physical help, needed
	Stairs	Ability to walk up and down the number of stairs needed for home independence; and the aids, verbal or physical help, needed
Self-care	Dressing	Ability to dress and undress; and the aids, verbal or physical help, needed
	Bathing	Ability to put bath plug in, turn water taps on and off and test water temp.; and the aids, verbal or physical help, needed
	Washing	Ability to wash face and hands, to shave, comb hair; and the aids, verbal or physical help, needed
	Toiletting	Able to clean self with toilet paper; and the aids, verbal or physical help, needed
	Eating and drinking	Ability to eat and drink; and the aids, verbal or physical help, needed
	Shopping	Ability to budget, use money, understand prices and check, or not, change given
	Cooking	Ability to make a cup of tea, snack or meal; and the aids and physical assistance needed
	Cleaning	Ability to dust, hoover and generally clean around the house; and the aids, verbal and physical help, needed

with patients is mainly during the day time, as abilities at night can be quite different. Darkness, drowsiness from sleep or medication, temperature change from warm bed to cold room, and postural change from lying to standing can all combine to make night time a risk period. Rolling in bed for Parkinsonian patients may prevent pressure sores, and access to toilet or commode prevent incontinence and degradation. All must be checked.

CONCLUSIONS FROM THE ASSESSMENT

The assessment of social, mental and physical functioning of the patient will give a clear idea of the present state, the desired state and what intervention is necessary to achieve it. It should also show if the patient has reached optimal functioning and so no longer needs help, or has deteriorated and needs re-assessment. The type of assistance required, such as aids and appliances, verbal prompting or physical assistance, can also be identified. The amount of assistance required and whether that level is available at home can be identified and extra help provided. It should also be borne in mind that over-helpful relatives can cause patients a disservice by decreasing their independence and tactful explanation is needed to prevent a disaster occurring.

Patients returning home to be on their own may need social stimulation to encourage them to maintain their appearance, hygiene and standards — few, of any age, would maintain high standards if no-one was likely to call, or there was nowhere to go.

The initial assessment will be used to form aims and objectives which are used to clarify the treatment programme required. This should always be explained to the patient so that he knows the reasons for the treatment and what is being required of him. Elderly people perform less well on tasks they feel have less meaning and they do not understand the relevance of.

When the initial stages have been accomplished there is a need for re-assessment. This will show if the patient has changed (either way) and whether the treatment programme needs to be changed accordingly. Each treatment should commence with an assessment of the patient and conclude with details of the session being recorded. Significant details should be discussed with the team.

SUMMARY

Assessment of the abilities and disabilities of the older patient is essential for realistic intervention, appropriate placement, and evaluation of change. Social, mental and physical aspects must be considered, as also must the reason for admission. The ability of the assessor and patient to communicate with each other is essential for success and any barriers found to exist must be eliminated. The social skills of the assessor will not go unrewarded. The assessment must take place in a conducive environment and the needs of the patient both during the assessment and the hospital stay, and any projection regarding his future, must be considered. Various activities to assist in socialisation — hopefully leading to a positive response to intervention — should be available for staff to use. As with all dealings with elderly people the subject is complex with much overlap between professions. Communication is the key to success.

REFERENCES

Beswick, K.B.J. (1987) Today there's none so deaf as can't be helped. *Geriatric Medicine, 17.5*, 55–77

Boardman, A.P. and Davenport, P. (1982) *A Guide to Assessment*. New Cross Hospital, London. (Available from the editors)

Challis, D.J. (1981) The measure of outcome in social care of the elderly. *Journal of Social Policy, 10*, 179–208

Hall, M.P.R. (1976) The assessment of disability in the geriatric patient. *Rheumatology and Rehabilitation, 15.2*, 59–63

Hodkinson, H.M. and Hodkinson, I. (1980) The influence of route of admission on outcome in the geriatric patient. *Age & Ageing, 9*, 229–34

Millard, P. (1982) Too much medicine, not enough care. *Health Service, 14*, 61–5

Murphy, E. (1986) *Dementia and Mental Illness in the Old*. Macmillan Papermac, London

Nicholls, P.J.R. (1976) Are ADL indices of any value? *British Journal of Occupational Therapy, 6*, 160–3

Quinn, J.L. and Ryan, N.E. (1979) Assessment of the older adult. *Journal of Geriatric Nursing, 5*, 2, 13–18

Rogers, J.C. (1980) Advocacy — the key to assessing the older client. *Journal of Geriatric Nursing, 6*, 1, 33–6

Rubenstein, L. (1983) The clinical effectiveness of multidimensional geriatric assessment. *Journal of the American Geriatric Society, 31*, 12, 758–62

Rubenstein, L., Schairer, C., Wieland, G. and Kane, R. (1984) Systematic biases functional status assessment of elderly adults: Effects of different data sources. *Journal of Gerontology, 39*, 6, 686–91

Squires, A.J. (1986a) Physiotherapy assessment of the elderly patient. *Physiotherapy, 72*, 12, 617–20

Squires, A.J. (1986b) Evolution of a specialty. *Therapy Weekly. 12*, 5–6, 31

Squires, A.J., Dolbear, R., Williams, R. and Smoker, S. (1987) Evaluation of Physiotherapy in a Day Unit. *Physiotherapy, 73*, 596–8

Therapy Weekly (1987) OT's Chair Clinic. *13*, 47, 16

Turnbull, P. (1982) *A Guide to the introduction of a personalised clothing service*. Disabled Living Foundation, London

5

Mental State and Physical Performance

Rosemary Oddy and Madeline Taylor

INTRODUCTION

The relationship between mental state and physical performance is apparent in many spheres of life. The athlete who requires his body to be at peak performance, needs to be able to push himself to the limits. His training equips him both physically and mentally so that he can combine strength, speed and ease of movement with the vital determination to win. The snooker champion's steady hand can be seen in close-up on the television screen, but this superb demonstration of co-ordination depends a great deal on his ability to maintain a calm and relaxed state of mind — sometimes aided by Beta-blockers!

Those who work in a stressful environment and have a demanding job are encouraged to indulge in some physical activity in order to 'wind down' at the end of the day. Running, walking, swimming, weight-lifting or whatever, exercise the body and increase the general well-being, as well as renewing mental energy and drive. The ability to relax, mentally and physically, can be learned; it can be of great benefit to those who are subjected to worries and stress, whether at examination time or during the course of a busy life.

The link between mental state and physical performance can be seen even more clearly amongst the mentally ill. Elderly patients who develop a major psychiatric condition may well be rendered incapable of carrying out the activities of daily living for a period of time; some, sadly, become permanently dependent on others. The intervention of occupational therapists and physiotherapists is particularly highlighted in this chapter but all team members, professional and lay, must work together following agreed aims and procedures to produce an effective result.

MENTAL STATUS TESTS AND RATING SCALES

It is possible to measure the extent of the patient's problems, since tests are available for this purpose.

There are many different types of tests in use in hospitals and clinics. Each location may favour particular ones that are considered to be more appropriate than others to the needs of the patient. The psychologist or doctor usually carries out the more intricate and time-consuming tests, but the nursing staff or other personnel may well complete a simple test with the patient.

Tests are used selectively and are carried out for a specific purpose. For example, information about the state of the patient's memory can be obtained from Hodkinson's ten-question mental test (Hodkinson 1972) and cognitive function can be tested via the Kendrick Battery (Gibson and Kendrick 1979). It is not appropriate to begin to describe these tests in details; it is preferable for team members to obtain further information on the tests used locally from their psychology department. However, an example of a simple memory/orientation test is included later on in the chapter, since it can form part of the therapist's own assessment procedure.

From the results of tests, the therapist will be able to gain a general impression of the patient's mental state and a relatively clear idea of what the patient might be able to achieve. Further information will be obtained less formally, from the assessment of the patient's response to group activities and from ADL. The areas of ADL which are given consideration are reading, listening to the radio, watching the television, writing, going out and hobbies. The functional activities assessed include shopping, cooking, cleaning, laundry, mobility (walking, stairs, transfers, moving on and off the bed), bathing, dressing, eating and drinking. The measuring scale, known as the Index of Independence of ADL (Katz and Akpom 1976) can be used to grade patients according to the level of their physical performance in a series of 'everyday' tasks. It encompasses the complex activities of bathing, dressing, toileting and transfer and the more basic ones of continence and feeding. These six functions are considered by Katz and Akpom to be hierarchically related in the order mentioned. The results of the Index serve as a guide to progress during therapy and are particularly useful when the future placement of the patient is under discussion. The precise levels of assistance needed by the patient are recorded, enabling the level on the classification scale to be established.

As far as elderly people with mental illness are concerned, there is a demonstrable link between their poor physical performance and their mental state. In both depression and dementia, functional mobility and independence in ADL may be severely affected, but as a result of quite different mechanisms (these will be described later). To further complicate the picture, multiple pathology is common in old age; joint stiffness, muscle weakness, the effects of drugs and limited exercise tolerance, for example, will additionally influence the level of the patient's performance and ADL. The rehabilitation of an immobile elderly patient suffering from a severe depression or dementia takes time, patience and ingenuity. The individual needs of each patient must be carefully considered at all stages of assessment and therapy. The plan of treatment should be discussed with and agreed by the patient whenever possible, and it should be realistic.

TRAINING FOR CARERS

It is expected that in the United Kingdom the enormous rise in the numbers of those aged 85 years and over will continue well into the twenty-first century; increasing from 569,000 in 1981 to 920,000 in 2011. The numbers of those aged 65 years and over will also continue to rise until 1991, but will then decrease (Coni et al. 1984). A proportion of those over 65 years will develop a mental disorder severe enough to require admission to hospital for care or treatment. One detailed study (Kay et al. 1964) found that 8 per cent of the elderly population in Newcastle-upon-Tyne were admitted to hospital suffering from a psychiatric disorder. Severe organic syndromes, mainly dementias, accounted for 5 per cent and severe major functional disorders for 3 per cent.

In the United Kingdom the future emphasis of care is to be in the community. So with a national policy of maintaining elderly mentally infirm (EMI) patients in the community, it is obvious that there will be an increasing need to support and train their carers, in addition to treating the patients themselves. Supporting the carers of those with dementia will require a whole range of services (Lodge 1981).

Frequently the main carer in a patient's home is the home help, who has built up a very close relationship over a period of time. In some areas of the United Kingdom (e.g. Darlington), the role of the home help has been extended to include simple but essential aspects of physical care of the patient, over and above the accepted domestic tasks (Stone 1986). This new breed of carer receives a basic training with an additional input provided by appropriate professional workers. The occupational therapist and the physiotherapist both play a significant part in the scheme by assessing the needs of the patient and then by giving the carer advice and training as required. In the future, therapists are likely to encounter many such innovative schemes set up in the community in an endeavour to assist the client, ease the task of carers and make the best use of scarce professional resources (Social Work Service Development Group Project 1984).

MAJOR MENTAL DISORDERS IN ELDERLY PATIENTS

Roth (1955) described the categories and incidence of mental disorders in the elderly. He considered that the acute confusional state, depression, paraphrenia and dementia were the four major disorders. Most medical practitioners consider the conditions in this particular order when making the diagnosis. By so doing, overuse of the unfortunate 'dementia' label is avoided, since consideration is given to the other three disorders first.

As an introduction, a brief outline only of these four conditions follows. No attempt is made to include all the symptoms of each condition, but rather to highlight those which particularly involve therapists.

An acute confusional state

This can arise as a result of any acute physical illness, but it is reversible if the underlying cause is treated. It can be precipitated by toxins produced by certain drugs or follow a sudden change in the normal pattern of life, such as death or a move of home. The physiotherapist attempting to treat such a patient, with an acute confusional state caused by a severe chest infection, may well find that the level of distress and excitability is such that little or no therapy can be carried out.

Depression

One of the most common mental disorders of the elderly, depression occurs more often in women than in men. This disorder, characterised by an abnormally lowered mood, may develop over a period of weeks or months. The patient shows a loss of interest in life and neglects his personal hygiene and appearance. He finds it difficult if not impossible to make decisions and to carry out essential daily activities; he may feel frustrated as a result and treats those around him with agression and hostility. Sleep and appetite are frequently disturbed, with a consequent loss of weight and lack of energy. Intelligence is not affected, although poor concentration and memory may give the false impression that it is; memory usually improves as the depression lifts. It is often the suicide risk or the inability to cope with everyday life which necessitates admission to hospital.

During the treatment period in hospital, anti-depressant drugs are taken by the patient. In some cases where the condition does not respond to drug therapy or if the depression is particularly severe, electro-convulsive therapy (ECT) may be given. This physical treatment remains controversial but can make an almost magical difference when applied to carefully selected patients. Therapists are likely to be involved with treating the patient's mental and physical problems. (This intervention will be described later.)

Paraphrenia

A less common mental illness, paraphrenia tends to affect women more than men. It is thought to be a form of schizophrenia which arises for the first time in those who are over the age of 60 years. The main symptoms are paranoid delusions, with the false ideas so firmly fixed in the patient's mind that no amount of reasoning can alter them. The anxiety associated with the delusions may necessitate referral to a therapist.

Dementia

An organic condition which involves brain cell loss, dementia leads to a progressive impairment of intellectual capacity.

There are two main types — senile dementia (Alzheimer's type) and multi-infarct (arterio-sclerotic) dementia. Senile dementia mainly affects women and results in a steady decline in ability. With multi-infarct dementia there is a characteristic step-like deterioration due to a series of mini-strokes; men being more commonly affected than women. The so-called pre-senile dementias occur before the age of 65 years and include Alzheimer's disease and Huntington's Chorea. Pick's disease and Jakob-Creuzfeldt disease are much rarer forms.

Dementia patients often pose many difficult management problems and can become very different people with profound personality changes. The short-term memory is commonly affected in varying degrees of severity and the patient becomes increasingly disorientated in time, place and person. The long-term memory, on the other hand, remains remarkably intact until the later stages of the disease. If the patient retains enough insight and is aware of these deficiencies, depression may well accompany the dementia. Communicating with the patient becomes a major problem; there may be expressive as well as receptive dysphasia. The misinterpretation of other people's actions or intentions can result in unexpected outbursts of aggression, whilst the inability to interpret the surroundings may provoke anxiety and fear. Mobility problems develop as the dementia progresses and walking and general mobility become impaired. Balance is affected and falls are frequent occurrences. Self-care skills also decrease, until bathing, dressing, toileting and, finally, feeding need full assistance.

An excellent booklet *Caring for the person with dementia* can be obtained from the Alzheimer's Disease Society (see Useful Addresses).

PREDICTING THE OUTCOME OF THERAPY

Therapists expect to encounter the more severe cases of depression and dementia in hospital and the less severe ones at home. However, many devoted carers (often a daughter) manage to support surprisingly incapacitated patients with dementia at home.

Dementia

In spite of the progressive nature of dementia and the fact that it is not curable, much can be done to ease the patient's problems and those of their carers. Therapy may be a concentrated session with the patient daily, but the outcome may depend upon how much additional practice can be incorporated into the rest of the day by carers and other members of the team. This applies whether the patient is at home or in hospital. A united approach is required.

A minor illness such as a common cold may be enough to upset the fragile balance between ability and inability and causes the dementia patient to go 'off his feet'. This does not necessarily mean that his walking days are over. Even after a bout of bronchopneumonia, the previous level of mobility can often be re-established with an encouraging approach and a very gradual re-introduction of functional activities and walking. A similarly positive attitude can be adopted towards the recovery expected following fractures and small strokes, although each incident must inevitably result in some loss of ability. There are, however, some dementia patients who do not respond well to therapy. Amongst them are those who refuse to co-operate in spite of all efforts and inducements, those whose memory is so badly affected that they are unable to retain an instruction long enough to carry it out, and those who show extreme sensitivity to pain following a fracture.

Depression

The eventual outcome for the severely depressed patient with mobility and self-care problems is generally good. The period of time involved may be long and is linked to the lifting of the depression. The patient's physical performance and mental state should be expected to return eventually near to that which existed prior to the depressive illness.

PARTICULAR POINTS TO CONSIDER DURING ASSESSMENT

The assessment is carried out on the lines described in an earlier chapter. There are, however, particular points which need to be considered or observed when assessing patients with dementia or depression.

The timing of the assessment can affect the results. Greater accuracy is likely if the activity to be tested is carried out at the

85

appropriate time of day. The assessment of other activities, which are not restricted to particular times, such as toileting and walking also need special considerations since the level of the performance may vary during the day. Therapists should visit the patient at different times in order to observe the extent of these fluctuations.

The assessment procedure may take several visits before it is completed. In the case of patients whose performance is severely affected by their psychiatric condition, it is important not to attempt too many tasks at one time and to ensure, with careful planning, that some measure of success is achieved. The patient should be allowed to finish on a high note.

As assessment carried out in the hospital can only reflect the patient's performance at that time and in that place. However, if the patient is to be discharged home or is at home, the most appropriate assessment is, of course, the one that is carried out there. Surrounded by familiar possessions, using his own well-known equipment and following his usual routine, the patient will demonstrate a much more reliable result.

The initial approach is particularly important and should not be rushed. The therapist must be quietly reassuring, but must also not overwhelm the patient by talking too much. A courteous greeting makes a good beginning, combined with the therapist's undivided attention. It is wise to use the patient's surname initially, unless requested otherwise; elderly people are, on the whole, unaccustomed to the current tendency to address virtual strangers by their forenames and can be upset by it. Self-esteem, already low in a depressed patient, may receive a boost with this simple demonstration of respect.

Dementia patients

Dementia patients frequently have difficulty in locating the source of sound or speech, therefore by addressing them by name, the problem is minimised. Very clear and concise explanations are always given so that the patient has the best opportunity of understanding. In some cases, the therapist may judge that the patient is unlikely to understand, but nevertheless gives him the benefit of the doubt and addresses him as if he does. It is unwise to talk about the patient within his hearing, or to appear to be discussing him from a distance; great discretion is required. Non-verbal communication is particularly effective with dementia patients so therapists should exploit the use of a friendly facial expression, a non-threatening body posture and a caring reassuring use of touch.

The dementia patient may be upset following admission and may require a couple of days in which to settle down before assessment is attempted. A multi-infarct dementia patient can be expected to show particularly well-defined variations in mood and physical performance from hour-to-hour, as well as from day-to-day.

The results of more than one assessment are required in order for a realistic report to be prepared. Three repetitions make it possible for the therapist to refer to the worst and the best performances when summarising findings. The report should clearly indicate the level of assistance required for each task, so that misunderstandings do not occur. There is a considerable difference between significant physical help and verbal guidance. In both cases one person is occupied with the patient for approximately the same length of time, but a strong healthy assistant is needed in one case and not in the other.

Multidisciplinary decisions regarding the possible placement of the patient are usually made as a result of the combined assessments of several agencies, including nurses, psychologists, occupational therapists, and physiotherapists.

Depressed patients

A depressed patient may show a great lack of interest and concentration and can give the erroneous impression that he does not understand what is being asked of him. Therapists need to remind themselves that in spite of this lack of response, the patient's intellect is not affected even if memory is temporarily impaired. A low-key approach is required and the therapist must give the patient time to express himself and must be ready to listen patiently to what he is saying. The reasons for the assessment are clearly explained to the patient, who may need to be gently persuaded to co-operate.

The patient's mood may well vary from day-to-day. Therefore, if he is obviously having an off-day it is best not to proceed with the assessment, but to return at another time.

Table 5.1: Twelve questions which form the information/orientation sub-test of the Cognitive Assessment Scale taken from the Clifton Assessment Procedures for the Elderly (Pattie and Gilleard 1979)

1	What's your name?
2	How old are you?
3	What is your date of birth?
4	What is this place/Where are you now?
5	What is your home address?
6	What is the name of this town/city?
7	Who is the Prime Minister?
8	Who is the President of the United States of America?
9	What are the colours of the British flag/Union Jack?
10	What day is it? NB NOT DATE
11	What month is it?
12	What year is it?

The number of correct answers are scored out of the possible 12. Patients with depression are expected to score 8 or more, whilst those with dementia are likely to achieve 7 or less

COGNITIVE ASSESSMENT TEST

If a simple memory test has not already been completed, a designated team member may carry it out as part of the assessment procedure (Table 5.1).

IDENTIFICATION OF PROBLEMS

A problem list is drawn up as a result of the assessment. Some problems can be avoided or lessened; sensory deficits are minimised simply by ensuring that any prescribed spectacles, hearing aids and dentures are in use if normally worn. Depersonalisation in hospital can also be decreased if arrangements can be made for patients to have a few possessions of their own around them and to wear their own clothes. In practice however, the use of the patients' own clothing is difficult to achieve since vast quantities may be needed and laundering and labelling can be a problem.

Footwear

The likelihood of falls is a problem met with in the care of elderly people and provision of footwear needs especial attention. More detailed information is given in Chapter 8, but the subject is also considered briefly here.

Falls can be caused if patients wear inappropriate footwear or slippers; the wearing of comfortable, well-fitting shoes increases stability and contributes to better balance. The foot is maintained firmly on the sole of the shoe instead of sliding off it, as so often happens when slippers are worn. An immediate improvement in the quality of gait can often be demonstrated. The height of the heel of the shoe can be an essential factor when compensation is needed for a tight tendo-calcaneus.

The increasing choice of acceptable washable shoes means that even the active but incontinent patient can be supplied with footwear. Sometimes, however, the sweating problem associated with man-made uppers may prevent their use. It is possible to protect leather shoes from the occasional incontinent episode with waterproofng liquid suitable for use on walking boots.

Access to a central stores which offers a choice of shoes suitable for elderly feet is a great asset; some psychiatric hospitals have such a facility. (The patients' clothing shop at Carlton Hayes Hospital, Leicester is one of the few laid out on the lines of a shop and funded by the NHS. It stocks a wide range of shoes and slippers as well as clothes. The clothing manager liaises with the physiotherapists and the chiropodist if particular fitting problems are encountered. An orthotist completes the team.)

There are many other problems specific either to depression or dementia which require treatment or management. These will be considered separately and details of the therapist's intervention will be given. The role of the physiotherapist with the elderly mentally ill is comprehensively discussed by Hare (1986).

THERAPY FOR PROBLEMS ASSOCIATED WITH DEPRESSION

The severity of the depression and the increasing inability to cope with the demands of everyday life bring the patient into hospital. Admission is also precipitated if there is a real risk of suicide. Therapy is directed towards the patient's state of mind and to his intellectual, social and functional problems.

The patient's self-esteem is low and he lacks confidence and motivation. He is therefore encouraged to participate in activities which can be easily achieved. Initially, simple tasks such as washing and drying dishes may be indicated in order to improve his morale. The level of difficulty of the activity chosen depends very much on the severity of the depression, with the more complex tasks being introduced as the patient's condition improves. There may be feelings of guilt and unworthiness, in which case individual counselling sessions may be appropriate. It is possible that suicidal threats may be voiced during therapy; they should always be taken seriously and reported immediately to nursing or medical staff. Participation in 'groups' gives the patient an opportunity to practise other skills. Quizzes, drama or other activity groups (Table 4.1) encourage the patient to communicate and exercise intellectual abilities, as well as improving social interaction. Relaxation training may be given for the anxiety which often accompanies the depression. The Mitchell Method of physiological relaxation (Mitchell 1971) is particularly easy for the patient to learn.

Hostility, aggression and lack of co-operation

A depressed patient often expresses intense anger and hostility towards those around him (Weissman *et al.* 1971). This stems from the frustration caused by his inability to function as before and because of his difficulty in communicating his real fears and worries. He may initially be uncooperative when asked to help on the ward or to attend a therapy session, not caring to face the fact that he is unable to carry out everyday tasks without assistance. If this occurs, the therapist waits a couple of days or until the medication takes effect before trying again. Then gentle coaxing may persuade him to participate in an activity, such as a cookery session, where there is an end-product. He is then able to give the cakes or biscuits to relatives or to other patients, boosting his self-esteem. Positive feedback in the form of praise enhances the likelihood of further co-operation. Other activities can then be introduced, beginning with the ones which the patient is known to enjoy. Gardening is often a favourite.

Patients may often show hostility or aggression towards staff or patients who try too hard to persuade them to join in. They are disinterested and lack confidence and concentration; they prefer to sit quietly and want to be left alone. The therapist may decide that for such a patient it is more appropriate for him just to sit and watch a group activity taking place. It is possible that at a later date his interest will be stimulated enough for him to find the confidence to join in with the other patients. This same patient may later feel guilty about his aggressive behaviour and will need to be reassured by the therapist that no offence was caused by it.

Disappointment can also cause aggression. This can best be avoided by always suggesting tasks which are well within the patient's physical and mental capabilities. The depressed patient feels vulnerable and needs plenty of sympathetic care. As the depression responds to treatment and the patient's condition improves, any inappropriate behaviour usually ceases.

A small proportion of patients develop very severe physical problems and become virtually immobile. There is often an underlying physical condition such as osteo-arthritis which is causing pain and stiffness. The patient complains of symptoms which he would normally tolerate well (Grimley Evans 1986). Some local physiotherapy may be given to help relieve the pain, and is usually most effective if carried out in conjunction with the essential active rehabilitation.

Advice on positioning and appropriate seating is important both to avoid poor sitting posture and to enable the patient to rise from sitting as easily as possible. General exercise group sessions also make a valuable contribution and add variety to the programme.

Elderly depressed patients are particularly susceptible to other infections. An acute chest infection can quickly take them off their feet. A concerted team effort is needed to ensure that pressure sores (Norton *et al.* 1962) or soft-tissue contractures are not allowed to develop during this period.

When the patient is considered well enough physically and mentally, preparations are made for the return home. The occupational therapist may accompany the patient on several visits to his own home in order to ascertain whether he is able to complete essential household tasks in familiar surroundings. This is of particular importance if the patient is returning to live alone.

MANAGEMENT OF PROBLEMS ASSOCIATED WITH DEMENTIA

The extent of each problem varies from patient to patient, therefore the therapist is unlikely to be faced with the task of managing all of them, all of the time. The therapist's assessment highlights those which will require particular attention during therapy. The overall aim is to enable the patient to be as independent as possible.

Communication

Difficulties in communication are often a major problem in spite of using all the required aids. In order to get the message across to the patient it may be necessary to utilise written as well as verbal and non-verbal methods. Progress may depend a great deal on effective communication. The patient's difficulty in understanding may be further increased by his poor concentration; it is therefore often only possible to engage in short bursts of activity or participation, interspersed with rests or pauses. Communication is a two-way process so it is equally important to listen carefully to what the patient says and to make a determined effort to understand what he means. (The general approaches to communication are described in detail in Chapter 3.) Some additional ways of communicating with dementia patients are now suggested.

Giving instructions The patient needs time to understand, so 'priming' consisting of the well-spaced repetition of instructions before the response is required, is useful. Care is, however, needed with the instruction itself. A 'direct' request such as 'Stand up' is preferable to 'Can you stand up?' This 'indirect' question form invites the possibility of a 'No' response and is best avoided if the action required must take place. Phraseology used locally may be more readily understood by the patient than the words or expressions normally used by staff. Experimentation is worthwhile and can be rewarding. So the Leicestershire patient may respond to 'Hotch up' when seated on the edge of the bed, but not to 'Move up'.

A pictorial instruction 'Nose over knees' may succeed where 'Lean forwards' does not. Careful wording can often successfully elicit a sub-cortical response where direct instructions for the same sequence of movements may fail. 'Come and help me lay the table' encompasses standing up and walking across the room for the given purpose of laying the table. It relieves the patient of the need to consciously organise himself to rise to standing and then to walk, since both occur automatically with such an instruction.

Using 'cues' Communication can be enhanced by using cues. A gentle tapping on the back of an appropriately positioned patient who has been asked to stand up, gives the cue to the movement required; a similar tapping to the hips of a patient practising chair-to-chair transfers helps to indicate the direction of the turn which the hips must make. Sound cues made by smacking the seat of a chair or a pillow on the bed, attract the patient's attention and add considerably to his understanding of the spoken request. Visual cues to movement can be provided during sitting-to-standing practise when the patient, seated on a chair, is flanked by two assistants. In this 'unison standing' manoeuvre the two helpers leaning forwards in a deliberately exaggerated manner give the patient strong visual cues with the movement of their heads. The sitting down movement is facilitated in a similar fashion.

Many such cues can be devised to augment the verbal instruction, in order to encourage the required movement or activity.

Disorientation

Orientation problems cause distress to dementing patients and particularly to those who have some insight remaining. Reminiscence therapy which makes use of the patients' more intact long-term memory may help to bring them up to date with the present. Cards (see Useful Addresses) make excellent visual aids for this purpose and enable conversation to take place on such subjects as transport, shopping and weddings. Comparisons between past memories and the present reality are emphasised.

Reality Orientation (Rimmer 1982) is directed more towards the patient's short-term memory problems. When it is used in the 24-hour format by everyone in contact with the patient, constant reminders help to keep him in touch with what is going on around him. The techniques can be used by carers at home as well as by hospital personnel.

It is particularly important that the structure and order of a normal day is maintained; night and day reversal can occur. It is therefore essential to have a large clock with a traditional face positioned where it can be easily seen; a digital clock is unfamiliar to elderly people and therefore unacceptable. It is also helpful to have a notice on the wall at home giving the patient's name and address. In hospital, a reality orientation board showing various details such as the name of the hospital, the correct day and date, the weather and the season is useful.

A specific reality orientation treatment group is carried out in hospital and usually consists of sessions of not more than three-quarters of an hour, two to three times a week.

Memory problems

Undue memory loss makes it increasingly difficult for the patient to carry out ADL in the correct sequence. 'Cues' can once again help to minimise the problem. For example, the occupational therapist retraining the patient to dress himself, arranges the patient's clothes in a logical and familiar order so that cues to the sequence are provided. Carers are also encouraged to use the same method each time the patient dresses. The importance of reinforcing a particular pattern with frequent and identical repetition cannot be over-stressed. It is possible that the patient may forget what he is doing in mid-activity; he should be given the necessary prompts to help him accomplish the task in hand.

Aggression

Patients with dementia often show aggression and hostility to those around them. They may use verbal abuse in the form of shouting or swearing or show physical aggression by hitting out, kicking or spitting, etc. There are some situations which render this type of behaviour more likely: the newly-admitted patient experiencing increased disorientation as a result of strange surroundings; the state of anxiety induced by the late arrival of a meal or visitor; and any unexpected demands made on an unprepared patient, such as a summons to go for an X-ray or to see the dentist. Frequent explanations and reminders are needed both to reassure and to prepare the patient so that aggressive responses are avoided. The stability and reassurance of a well-structured day, such as that in a hospital, often seem to suit the needs of these patients.

The cause of the aggression is not always apparent, in which case a note needs to be made of occurrences immediately preceding the inappropriate behaviour. A pattern of trigger factors may emerge as a result of these recordings. These situations can then be avoided and better behaviour reinforced by spending time with the patient when he is not aggressive. The key-worker system (Sugden 1986), where a specific member of staff is allocated to each patient, gives the patient someone familiar to turn to when he feels anxious and frustrated.

Physically active dementia patients who like to wander at will often become restless and aggressive if space on the ward is limited and there is no access to an enclosed garden. The necessary freedom of movement can be achieved by taking such 'wanderers' for a long walk in the hospital grounds or to the local shops. Goodwin (1984) has suggested that 'wanderers' are those who stroll further than is comfortable to whoever is in charge!

Therapists can avoid provoking anxiety and aggression during therapy by giving the patients time to carry out the required activities at their own pace. Dysphasic patients may become frustrated by their inability to communicate and respond by lashing out. (Guidelines for dealing with dysphasia are covered in Chapter 3.)

Pain and fear These can also cause aggression. The patient who has fallen several times may understandably become afraid of falling when he moves. He may as a result refuse or be reluctant to leave the safe haven of his chair. He may also show great fear when being moved on the bed. Reassurance and very careful physical handling minimise the fear caused during manoeuvres on the bed. The use of a stout dining chair in front of the seated patient overcomes his reluctance to leave his chair. The dining chair placed with its back to the patient fills the space ahead and offers visual reassurance. It is important for the patient to rise to standing using a double arm thrust *before* holding onto the chair for support. Therapists can devise similar solutions for other fear-making situations and so avoid the possibility of aggression.

The physiotherapist is often faced with the necessity of carrying out movements which can cause pain, for example following fractures. Pain-killing drugs are usually necessary before treatment so that pain is reduced and an aggressive response is avoided. The progression of treatment following fractures often has to be unusually slow until the pain subsides.

An empathetic approach to the patient's fears and anxieties helps to minimise much of the aggression which might otherwise occur during therapy.

MISINTERPRETING THE ENVIRONMENT

Dementia patients are aware of their surroundings and can be profoundly affected by them. Jazzy patterns on a carpet may be taken for objects spilt on the floor and the patient tries to pick them up. A self-reflection in a mirror or window may be interpreted as an intruder and can cause great distress. A shaft of sunlight shining on the floor can bring the patient to a stop or cause him to walk over or round it. He may step very deliberately up and over a silver threshold strip or a long dark area of pattern on the flooring which he interprets as a step, landing heavily as a result of the misjudged action. This 'stepping-response' may upset the patient's balance and cause him to fall. When assisting a patient who shows such a response, firm and repeated reassurances should be given that the floor is flat; it is possible to maintain an uninterrupted rhythm of walking with such intervention. Carers should be encouraged to reassure the patient in similar situations, acting as an 'interpreter' of the surroundings on his behalf.

MOBILITY PROBLEMS

The therapist must manage the problems associated with the dementia whilst attempting to promote some useful functional mobility (Oddy 1987). Reference has already been made to the patient's possible reluctance to move as a result of fear or pain and to the difficulty in carrying out sequences of movements involving conscious organisation. The strategies for overcoming these and other problems were also suggested earlier, together with examples of some functional movements. More examples of exercises which might be used to encourage mobility are now given.

Retraining sitting to standing

The inability to rise from sitting into a supported standing position makes bathing, dressing and some aspects of care such as toileting difficult and time-consuming. If this problem can be overcome, albeit in easy stages, the carer and the patient will both benefit.

Initially, the patient may need to experience the shift of body weight from the hips to the feet, in preparation for the standing-up movement. This can be achieved when the therapist, seated on the edge of a low bed beside the patient, gently nudges him sideways. The patient responds by shifting his hips away from the therapist, using a double arm thrust against the bed to achieve the momentary transfer of weight through his feet. Afterwards 'unison standing', previously mentioned in the context of 'visual cues', can be used to facilitate the full movement of rising to standing. The use of a 'high perch' is also worth considering, since when seated on a raised surface, the patient is at such a mechanical advantage that standing up requires very little effort. An adjustable plinth or the padded arm of a stout dining chair may be suitable for this purpose. Transfers can, if necessary, be facilitated in a similar manner, by using two easy chairs with the addition of a second firm cushion in each to raise the height of their seats. Having successfully experienced the feel of the transfer movement several times, the same manoeuvre can be repeated without the extra cushions or with thinner ones. Patients who are afraid of leaning forwards during the transfer often respond surprisingly well to a third stout chair placed in front of the two needed for the transfer. Once again the chair, used to fill the space in front of the patient, reassures him and gives him the confidence to carry out the movement.

Preparation for walking

Sometimes the patient manages to rise from sitting and then fails to stay upright because his knees buckle. It may then be worthwhile splinting one of the patient's legs to overcome this. By providing him with one comfortable rigid 'pillar' to stand on, he is able to experience the sensation of a more upright posture. He is also able to experiment safely with taking weight through the unsplinted leg. Reflexly joint compression and stimulation of the proprioceptors under the splint add their effects.

Before walking is attempted, it is desirable for the patient to be able to balance steadily and independently whilst holding onto a suitable support. Initially, additional support is required, but this should be carefully withdrawn as soon as possible so that the patient is encouraged to make a full contribution.

Walking aids The patient who is unsteady on his feet and lacks confidence often benefits from some form of mechanical support.

The walking aid selected needs to suit his individual requirements and the available space. Some patients are, however, unable to manoeuvre an aid in a confined space and prefer to use the furniture for support. A piece of equipment which can be pushed across the floor is likely to be more suitable than a frame but is sometimes less easy to use on a thick carpet. The type which has a braking system incorporated into its two front wheels (e.g. mobilator or rollator) is the simplest and safest to use. A walking stick is occasionally helpful but is frequently viewed with anxiety in residential homes and hospitals because of its potential as a weapon!

Retraining other aspects of mobility

Other mobility problems, including the inability to get on and off the bed and to move on the bed are retrained in a similar manner. The patient is initially given the 'feel' of the movement, which may if necessary be carried out passively; it may need to be repeated several times, before he can be expected to contribute to the movement. The movement is then practised with assistance, which is gradually reduced over a period of time. Eventually it is hoped that the patient will be able to complete the movement with verbal guidance and the use of cues only or, better still, unaided.

Rigidity often hampers the patient's ability to move. The carer also has great difficulty in assisting him because of the awkwardness of his board-like body. Rhythmical trunk rotations given whilst the patient is lying down or in a sitting position are usually most effective in temporarily reducing the rigidity, so that he is able to move more freely afterwards.

Individual sessions are essential for specific retraining, but group exercises offer valuable opportunities for additional stimulation. They enable variety to be introduced into the programme and are useful for maintenance purposes. Gratifying results are often obtained spontaneously, especially when music is used. The group sessions should of course be enjoyable.

PROBLEMS WITH ADL

The importance of maintaining the normal order and structure of the day as far as possible has already been stated. The need to practise tasks at the relevant time of day has also been discussed. The patient is much more likely to complete a task successfully when using familiar equipment, with old habitually employed methods in familiar surroundings.

Retraining

If the patient is unable to carry out the task unaided, verbal prompting or assistance is given to ensure its smooth completion. It may be necessary for the therapist to carefully demonstrate the sequence to the patient, as for example during a cookery session, or to carry out others, such as shaving or teeth-cleaning, on the patient himself. Repetition and regular practice facilitate the tasks.

Domestic and household chores, together with self-care activities are complex in nature and consist of skills which have been learnt and perfected over many years. Most of these activities involve the necessity to carry out each stage in a particular order, something which dementia patients find increasingly difficult. The decline in intellectual processes and memory tend gradually to deprive the patient of his ability to care for himself.

Minimising problems

There are many simple ways of minimising the patient's difficulties. A few examples are now described.

Feeding aids These are particularly effective. For example, the non-slip Dycem mat which prevents the patient's plate from travelling across the table; the plate-guard which keeps the food on the plate; and the non-spill feeder which can be managed by the patient when the use of a cup becomes impracticable.

Planning The complicated process of making a cup of tea and dressing is eased if the items to be used are laid out in a logical order beforehand. Unnecessary problems can be avoided by selecting items of clothing for the patient's wardrobe which have manageable fastenings.

Supervision Bathing needs supervision for safety reasons. It can nevertheless become a very frightening experience for the patient, who may be unable to control his balance whilst in the water. An overhead shower is not considered to be a good alternative for an elderly patient who is not accustomed to one, but a hand-held shower used while the patient sits in the bath is usually acceptable. A non-slip mat in the base of the bath is advisable.

Encouraging activity at home

The dementia patient who is being maintained at home may need a great deal of community support. Input from the Home Help Service and Meals-on-Wheels eases some problems. Regular monitoring should be provided by the community psychiatric nurse, social worker or therapist and co-operation of the relatives and willing neighbours should be encouraged.

The patient may not be able to carry out the normal complex household and domestic chores, but the therapist encourages him to remain active in the home. There are some easy tasks which a female patient enjoys doing, probably badly, but nevertheless they occupy the patient's time (e.g. dusting, sweeping, arranging flowers and hand-washing). A male patient often enjoys pottering in the garden. It will be interesting to note if future 'liberated' generations return to traditional gender responsibility tasks.

A discreet explanation to the local shop-keeper and the post office clerk about the patient's difficulty in handling money may be a wise move, if the patient is to be encouraged to continue shopping and collecting his weekly pension. The occupational therapist advises the carers what tasks the patient can reasonably be expected to do.

SUMMARY

The mental state and physical function of elderly patients are very much interlinked. An examination of the problems associated with depression or dementia highlight this situation. However, the content and scope of the programme of activities selected for the patient with depression is very different from the one required by the patient with dementia. The clinically-depressed patient is expected to make a good recovery; the low mood gradually lifts with treatment and normal function is usually restored. The dementia patient does not recover; his intellectual capability slowly declines and his physical functioning deteriorates. Therapy helps the patient to retain a degree of independence for as long as possible.

Therapists have a significant role to play in the multidisciplinary team involved in the mental and physical care of these elderly patients and in the support of their carers.

REFERENCES

Coni, N., Davison, W.I. and Webster, S. (1984) *Ageing: the Facts*. Oxford University Press, Oxford

Gibson, A.J. and Kendrick, D.C. (1979) *The Kendrick Battery for the Detection of Dementia in the Elderly*. NFER Publishing Co., Windsor, Ont

Goodwin, S. (1984) On desolation row. *New Age* (Autumn), 22–7

Grimley Evans, J. (1986) The interaction between physical and psychiatric disease in the elderly. *Update* (February), 265–70

Hare, M. (1986) *Physiotherapy in Psychiatry*. Heinemann, London, pp. 66–93

Hodkinson, H.M. (1972) Evaluation of a mental test score for assessment of mental impairment in the elderly. *Age and Ageing, 1*, 233–8

Katz, S. and Akpom, C.A. (1976) A measure of primary sociobiological function. *International Journal of Health Services, 6*, No. 3, 493–508

Kay, D.W.K., Beamish, P., and Roth, M. (1964) Old age mental disorders in Newcastle-upon-Tyne. *British Journal of Psychiatry, 110*, 146–58

Lodge, B. (1981) *Coping with Caring*. MIND, London, 28–34

Mitchell, L. (1971) *Simple Relaxation*. Murray, London

Norton, D., McLaren, R. and Exton-Smith, A. (1962) Pressure sores. In *Investigation into Geriatric Nursing Problems*, National Corporation for the Care of Old People, 193–238

Oddy, R.J. (1987) Promoting mobility in patients with dementia: some suggested strategies for physiotherapists. *Physiotherapy Practice, 3*, No. 1, 18–28

Pattie, A.H. and Gilleard, C.J. (1979) *Manual of the Clifton Assessment Procedures for the Elderly (CAPE)*. Hodder and Stoughton Educational, Sevenoaks

Rimmer, L. (1982) *Reality Orientation: Principles and Practice*. Winslow Press, Buckinghamshire

Roth, M. (1955) The natural history of mental disorder in old age. *Journal of Mental Science, 101*, 281–301

Social Work Service Development Group Project (1984) *Supporting the Informal Carer 'Fifty Styles of Caring'*, DHSS, London

Stone, M. (1986) Keeping care at home. *Health Services Journal*, 730

Sugden, J. (1986) The nurse's role in the Therapeutic team. In *A Handbook for Psychiatric Nurses*. Harper and Row, London, 25–7

Weissman, M.M., Klerman, G.L. and Paykel, E.S. (1971) Clinical evaluation of hostility in depression. In G.C. Davison and J.M. Neale, *Abnormal psychology*, 4th edition. Wiley, New York

6

To Rehabilitate or Not?

Amanda Squires and Patricia Wardle

The assessment procedures already described in Chapters 4 and 5 will have identified the current abilities of the patient and compared them with both prior and desired ability to enable discharge to the preferred environment.

TEAM ROLE

The role of the team is now to identify the intervening gap and assess the realistic form and quantity of intervention, if any, to be employed. Aspects such as prognosis, resources, motivation, unit policy and abilities of carers are amongst the items to be considered by team members, including the patient and relatives. Communication between team members is essential as is an appreciation of the difficulties each may confront in his or her task. Not all elderly patients are medically or psychologically suitable for rehabilitation and not all professionals can provide an across the board service irrespective of a patient's desire or response. Selection of priorities is a hard choice but we hope the following will help to make the decisions easier to make.

Prognosis

The prognosis of the patient's medical condition elicited by the doctor must be shared with the rest of the team, as must the physical, mental and social prognosis from other team members. In terms of physical performance, similar patients with 'identical' strokes may present, but on assessment it may be found that for one it is the first event in a previously active and healthy life, and for the other one of a series in a housebound life accompanied by mental deterioration. The aims for both will be quite different, but must also be clear to all involved. The impact of the stroke on the patient and relatives will also be quite different, probably much more devastating to the first.

Resources

Physical and material resources will never meet the increasing demands being put upon them by an ageing population and prioritisation is a necessity. Unfortunately, the wants of the patient may exceed the needs and a basic level of independence may have to be the goal. Delegation of tasks to unqualified staff can be considered where appropriate, and the importance of including relatives and carers in the patient's rehabilitation is a largely untapped resource probably emanating from reserve and exaggerated anxiety on both sides. The use of volunteers to undertake tasks which would otherwise not have been possible, to tie in with local Trade Union agreements, can also be considered.

Material resources such as treatment modes, aids and appliances must meet the needs of the individual situation. Many items available on the market for the general public are ideally suited for assisting disabled people of all ages and are therefore less expensive and more acceptable than 'special' items. The remote-control television is a good example and if elderly and disabled people were considered fully when plans are drawn up for buildings, furniture and fittings, the need for specialist items would be considerably decreased. Before supplying any aid or appliance, several basic questions should be asked:

(i) Is it essential or is it a 'gift'?
(ii) Has the patient already got one or something similar?
(iii) Do they know how to use it or can they be taught?
(iv) Will they use it and how can you check?
(v) Is it essential for the home situation?

The classic story of the patient immobile because of the large number of walking aids, 'one from each admission', restricting his space is so common as to be an embarrassment. It is estimated that up to 60 per cent of aids supplied are not used, depending on the type (Grant 1985). Increasing disability after issue of an aid may cause non-use, and there is also lack of awareness as to how discarded aids can be returned which should alert the resource-conscious into action to consider a retrieval system.

Motivation

Hesse and Campion (1983) confirm what many frequently think: that 'one of the most frustrating experiences in geriatric medicine is caring for the patient who has the physical capacity for rehabilitation but lacks the motivation to participate in a rehabilitation programme'. Blaming failure on the patient is an easy answer, but does not solve the problem. Rehabilitation is at its most demanding when response is required of the patient, and the therapist cannot do it for him (e.g. coughing). Suchett-Kaye *et al.* (1971) found that lack of motivation appeared to be an important bar to progress in rehabilitation.

For the patient to be motivated to respond the purpose of the activity must be relevant and some success in the activity anticipated. Explanation as to why the neck is being examined when the patient came with finger tingling may seem unnecessary to the examiner, but essential to the patient if he is to have any confidence in the ability of the assessor. One of the biggest barriers to motivation is a confused team where information and aims from different members may differ or even oppose each other. Motivation of the team is also an important factor and the patient will often echo the attitudes he finds.

We may also contribute to lack of motivation when we use as a 'goal' the last thing the patient wants. For example 'when you can walk you can go home', when at evening visiting the relatives are making it quite clear that home is no longer possible. The patient is put in an invidious position and is more likely to respond to family loyalty — but not always! Such pieces of information gleaned by team members must be reported to the relevant specialist so that the barriers to rehabilitation can be lifted by resolution of the problem.

Improvement in patient co-operation can also be made by paying attention to his basic needs. The 'Hierachy of need' proposed by Maslow (1954) is not always considered, and will do nothing but good.

(i) Basic physiological needs (e.g. eating, drinking, eliminating, dressing). No-one stands and walks if he fears incontinence or inadequate clothing cover.

(ii) Safety needs — has the patient confidence in you, the equipment, and the floor? Has he seen you allow another patient to fall?

(iii) Needs for affection ⎱ basic social skills
(iv) Needs for esteem ⎰ should achieve these

(v) Self-realisation — satisfaction with the tasks accomplished — does the patient know what the goal is and when he has achieved it?

Unit policy

There are as many policies as there are units and all team members must be aware of the rules under which they work. Bucking the system is for the missionary zeal of inexperience and usually achieves little. Some admission wards have a deadline of weeks or even days before patients are transferred to 'rehabilitation' or 'long-stay'. Some units admit patients and keep them on the same ward through all stages of rehabilitation, and re-admit them to the same ward should the need arise. Isaacs (1986) identified the phenomenon of 'Ultimately Immobile Patients' as those who had been hospitalised for at least three months and were unable to walk and transfer without human assistance. He found the greater number to be inversely proportional to admission rates and qualified nurse input.

There are advantages and disadvantages of all systems and enquiry into the reason for the policy may satisfy frustration. Policies are not written once for all time and can be reviewed as changes occur. Good reason, diplomatically presented, may produce the best response. Historical unwritten rules also exist and 'We've never done it like that before' is an opportunity for re-education and progress. Sensitivity is needed where staff are entrenched and may feel threatened by new ideas. Visits to other units or outside speakers may stimulate discussion and 'blame' for the new initiatives can be put outside rather than inside the unit.

Carers' abilities

Rubenstein *et al.* (1984) has identified that patients perceive their functioning at a higher level than the nurse or the carer. He suggests that denial of disability, optimism, recollection of prior ability, or concealment may be the explanation for the patient's view. An over-burdened carer may well exaggerate the disability of the patient to facilitate the provision of additional help. In addition, the patient may appear less able than has been identified due to hospital routine and inadequate communication.

Carers should also prove their stated abilities because presumption of an ability can often exceed its performance (Coates and King 1982). The ability and commitment of the carer should also be considered. 'My daughter is wonderful and will do anything for me' may not be reciprocated by the daughter who has other commitments, perhaps to other equally disabled relatives, and may also be of pensionable age herself. At a dependent level, the decision as to whether a patient remains in a long-stay facility or returns home may depend on a member of the family learning how to transfer the patient (Reed and Gessner 1979).

For some patients where prognosis is poor, the team must consider Tender Loving Care (TLC) as the intervention of choice, not as a failure but as the best choice for the patient. This will entail facilitating nursing care by the provision of suitable furniture and aids, prevention of contractures and pressure areas, appropriate measures for faecal and urinary continence, prevention or control of pain, and the relief of respiratory distress. The care provided for each area will depend on the team composition, but there must be overlap and an appreciation of the importance of the role of the nurse as co-ordinator.

There will be some patients for whom independence in even the smallest activity (such as drinking), will be important for the quality of their lives and this should be encouraged. Ransome (1978) suggested that 'every time someone does a movement for an elderly patient of which he is capable himself — another square inch of his long-stay bed is reserved'. When the patient's capabilities have been identified, this statement should be remembered.

QUALITY OR QUANTITY OF LIFE

Modern technology has the ability to prolong life, almost without the patient, but the old adage 'quality or quantity' must be considered. Attempts have been made to measure quality of life in health care, but Denham (1983) feels that there is no single universally accepted definition or measurement of 'quality of life'. The problem facing the professional is how best to use available resources, and calculations are unconciously being made in terms of the number of people with the problem, cost of intervention and follow-up care, and length of survival. Other factors are often added to this equation such as the social significance of intervention, experience of available staff, availability of resources at the time, etc. Guidex (1986) emphasises the importance of determining 'effectiveness' and describes the Quality Adjusted Life Year (QALY) where years in good health after a procedure (such as heart transplantation) can be calculated against years another patient with another procedure would describe as only 50 per cent in good health. The problem becomes very complex when older patients with poor prognosis still have to exist for the remainder of their lives as financially dependent on society. Stokes-Roberts (1986) reminds us that we are the elderly of the future, and if we recognise our own needs, likes and dislikes we will see and understand many of those of our patients. Denham (1983) feels that assessment of physical and mental health, life satisfaction, morale, the environment and staff attitudes are the most useful measures. Aspects of these are described elsewhere. What remains essential is communication between staff so that changes in both the patient and the management routine are known and implemented (Rosenberg *et al.* 1986).

The final stage of life

Only when the team is convinced that active rehabilitation is inappropriate do the alternatives need to be looked at. It may be that the patient needs more to be helped to live the final days of his life with acceptance and contentment.

The whole of life from birth to death is a continuum and the point of death varies along that life line. These two factors, birth and death, are the only two certainties in our lives.

Elderly patients and death

For some elderly patients death comes as a welcome friend, one with whom they are familiar for they were born in an age when infant mortality was high, when death in childbirth was commonplace, when there were no antibiotics or sulphonamides. Death therefore was familiar in natural circumstances. Add to that the fact of two world wars, and countless others in which the Western world has been involved, and one will see that elderly patients have not been protected from the ravages of death and the natural accompanying grief as have the present generation, growing up in the 1980s.

Therefore, in regarding the elderly patient and death we need to be aware that our own experience and feelings about death may be different from that of our elderly patients. Another consideration will be that few of their friends and relatives of contemporary age are still alive and so the prospect of death may not be so threatening for these patients as for younger people. They will also know that, in the main, their own families are not dependent upon them so that to face death is something they can do without the dependency ties and worries a younger person may have.

Facing death

How then do elderly people face death? The answer is with many varying attitudes. Some will feel cheated because they have not reached the age they hoped for, or their parents achieved, others will hope to be the second of a marriage partnership to die, only to find they are the first to face death.

Elderly people will experience the same feelings as anyone who faces death. These are recognised as Denial, Anger, Bargaining, Depression, Acceptance (DABDA).

Similar feelings will be experienced by those who grieve and those who care for people who cannot be rehabilitated. One of the most difficult feelings to cope with is helplessness. This may be particularly difficult for therapists who usually are in the habit of helping, actively doing things and encouraging the patient towards rehabilitation. Suddenly to be faced with helplessness, and not to be needed can be very hard and the feeling needs to be recognised and owned by the therapist as do the feelings experienced by dying and bereaved people. We shall explore these now.

Denial Patients often react by denying the facts when told that no further help is available for them by saying that, despite what the doctor said, they feel better than last week; or patients will make a very determined effort to do something extra, to prove to themselves that whatever the doctor said they are not prepared to accept it at first, and rarely are they able to discuss their feelings at this stage apart from the denial of the truth.

Anger The patient may well want to lash out at the world that they are gradually leaving. Everyone may be considered to be against them and thus provoke anger. The anger may take the form of constant complaints about those who are caring for the patient, arousing memories of another unfairness in life. It may be directed against the medical profession in general, of whom the therapists are a part, as the patient may well believe he has had a bad deal.

Bargaining The next stage is often one of bargaining, hoping that death can be deferred for a while. Special family events can help here, the expected new grandchild, or a wedding may give the patient ground to hold onto life until attendance at that special event has been achieved. There is likely to be some 'if only' statements. 'If only the doctor had come sooner, or my family had realised I was ill . . .' 'If only I could be at home/visit my son once more . . .'

Depression The fourth characteristic of the patient realising that death is approaching is the feeling of depression. Nothing seems worth bothering about and during this stage all communication with the patient may be extremely difficult. Body and eye contact may be avoided at all costs and a feeling of resignation may well take the place of the normal verbal response which will be recognised by those who care for the patient.

Acceptance This stage of dying may be reached at various times depending upon the previous experiences of the patient, and their actual medical condition and their own self-understanding. The patient will be able, and indeed may want to share his feelings about dying. There will be a sense of loss and letting go. There will be sadness perhaps at not seeing grandchildren and great grandchildren reach maturity. The sadness may also be related to the actual fact that life has been very good and the patient may not want to let it go. On the other hand many patients who are elderly will welcome the relief that dying brings to them because they may be very tired with the struggle to maintain a reasonable quality of life.

In letting go the responsibility to live, many elderly people are able to die with the dignity they want as long as physically and emotionally they can be kept as comfortable and pain-free as possible. They will consider they have had a very good life and they are quite ready to let it go and indeed are able to help medical staff and therapists come to terms with their own feelings about death and about patients dying.

CARERS HAVE FEELINGS TOO

Professional carers are, of course, owners of feelings and the feelings associated with grief are no exception.

Consider the case where a team has seen great potential for rehabilitation in an elderly patient and short-term and long-term aims have been achieved, to a point where a patient is due to be discharged home to a very acceptable quality of life. Then death comes. Relatives, medical staff and therapists will experience the same feelings as the dying patient (DABDA), and will have to learn to come to terms with those feelings and accept them to be free to help other patients.

The first reaction on being told of the death of a patient similar to the one given as an example above, will be to wonder if the identity of the deceased patient is accurate, or was it really a very ill patient who died. Anger may be felt in questions such as, 'Why did that patient have to die — the only real home rehabilitation patient I had.' Bargaining may be connected with statements which belie a 'no-win' situation for the therapist. 'If I had worked harder to clear the patient's chest he may not have died', counteracted with, 'If I had not made the patient work so hard their heart may not have been so strained and perhaps they would not have died.'

Staff may experience depression, not always realising that there is good reason for the feelings of flatness and despondency. Only in the light of all the feelings will the full acceptance of the patient's death be possible and that may also rouse feelings for team members about their own mortality, the mortality of those nearest to them, guilt and feelings of loss.

How staff learn to come to terms with these feelings for

themselves will determine the way they are able to help patients and their relatives. It is sometimes a new experience for a professional to allow other people to recognise their feelings, for they are trained to *do* things rather than *feel* things. The reality is that the two cannot be separated, but we can deny the feelings ourselves and to others.

The team will have to learn, often from more experienced people or in seeking professional help, how to care for themselves when the feelings related to death and grief are there. By recognition of such feelings, their own needs at the time and their willingness to recognise that they are not superhuman, carers will in turn be able to conduct themselves with sensitivity and remain able to care for their patients and their relatives. Each professional, too, will need to recognise that other members of the team may also be affected by grief and loss and may not be willing to easily admit it.

One of the difficulties is that professional carers, who spend years training to help people live and to be rehabilitated after illness and injury, frequently find it hard to realise that death can snatch a patient at a moment's notice and leave the carers with a lot of uncomfortable feelings. Therefore, staff will need to find a safety valve in order to release their feelings and thereby remain patient-centred, until death, or rehabilitation, is achieved.

The anxieties of patients, relatives and professionals can be resolved when all those involved are gently and firmly in full possession of the knowledge that death is not a vague possibility but is imminent and real. When a patient, his relatives and the team are clear that the imminent death will be with dignity and will be pain-free, a 'good death', then the acceptance of the truth will be possible. Openly and honestly working together can lead to a rich experience of death when no further rehabilitation is possible, or desirable.

This open, honest approach will allow time for recognition to be given to the ending of the relationship and for good-byes to be said among the patient, relatives, friends and carers. This is, then, a complete relationship followed through until its natural conclusion.

ACTIVE REHABILITATION

If, after consideration of the assessment findings, active rehabilitation is agreed as the option of choice, the long- and short-term aims must be quite clear to all participants (i.e. the ward team including ancillary staff, patient and carers), particularly bearing in mind the fact already referred to of the carer's view of the patient as 'helpless' in the hospital environment (Rubenstein *et al.* 1984). It should also be remembered that rehabilitation is a 24-hour process and any assistance required at any time during the day or night from any person or piece of equipment will need to be repeated in the community setting, and vice versa if a patient is admitted. It is so easy to cause further dependence by lack of thought. Again, team communication is essential.

SETTING OF AIMS

Long-term aims will be set by the team and, hopefully, will be to discharge the patient back to his own home. In the United Kingdom we are less accustomed to setting time-scales as well, but in the absence of hard data, experienced staff will rely on 'intuition and experience' to assist in this planning. The ultimate aim will be broken down into smaller goals; the involvement of the patient and carers in goal-setting and recognition of achievement is essential. Consistent approaches to intervention at all stages is vital, for instance if 'independent chair drill' is an aim, all members must encourage it, whether it is at the lunch table, during speech therapy or in visiting the toilet (Mort 1985). Obstacles to the attainment of each goal must be identified and overcome. Inability to get out of a chair can be caused by a multitude of factors such as:

 (i) Lack of communication (e.g. language, hearing, sight).
 (ii) Lack of understanding of task.
 (iii) Lack of motivation to comply.
 (iv) Structure of the chair.
 (v) Floor covering.
 (vi) Painful feet and inadequate footwear.
 (vii) Fear.

These factors are in addition to the more commonly assessed factors, such as power and joint range.

The actual barrier must be found, not the whole task recorded as 'cannot do'. The unfortunate aspect of rehabilitation is that frequently the patient is required to undertake the activity which may have caused the original referral (e.g. walking retraining when it was a fall when walking that caused the problem). Therefore, the patient's fear of a repeat performance must be appreciated and dealt with sensitively. Timor Cadenii, or the phobic fear of falling, is a problem very familiar to physiotherapists dealing with older patients. The patient typically sits leaning backwards in the chair gripping the arm rests and any attempt to get him to stand will result in the chair coming too. Familiarising the patient with the floor, by use of rolling and crawling exercises, will allow him to see that it can be got on to and up from. This will lessen his fear and will enable chair drill to be practised prior to walking retraining. The alternative, prising the patient out of the chair and 'walking him between two' with his feet experiencing dubious contact with the floor, does nothing positive for the patient and little for the status of the staff involved.

The provision of help in the initial stages of any activity is important for promoting confidence. Handling a disabled person is an acquired skill, which experienced staff may underrate. Techniques found suitable for individual patients need to be shared with the team, not kept a secret by the initiated.

- if no help is needed — don't provide it
- if one person is needed, use only one
- if two are needed, use two — but remember the patient is the reason for the paired activity, not staff news exchange!

FUNCTION, RANGE OR DIAGNOSIS?

In regard to older patients, controversy exists over what to assess and manage. All factors are important, but the relative importance of each can only be seen in the context of all the others. Nicholls (1976) suggests that it is in the chronic disorders and with old age that functions assume considerable importance. The relevance of treatment to the reinstatement of a function may also be more apparent to the patient, and Hesse and Campion (1983) have shown that elderly individuals perform less well on tasks that they feel have less meaning and that they do not understand the connection of. A patient with any diagnosis can manage at home provided that he and his carers can manage at least the basic functions of life.

Ability to perform the functions necessary for a maximally-independent life in the chosen environment must be the aim, and factors preventing this will need to be defined and dealt with, if appropriate, by the relevant team members, who must communicate and record their findings to enable a whole picture of problems and progress to be produced.

WHERE TO TREAT

By choice the patient's usual environment is the ideal venue for rehabilitation but social, medical and environmental factors may have caused him to be removed from it. Anywhere away from this environment is an artificial situation for physical, mental and social management if the aim is for independence at home. For instance, many elderly people are accustomed to slip mats, trailing electrical flexes, inadequate lighting and use of a gas oven as a main source of heat often irrespective of 'professional' advice. These surroundings replicated in hospital would certainly contravene the Health and Safety Act. The home environment may not only reflect the physical surroundings but also the usual lifestyle and social contacts the patient has. Wherever the treatment takes place it should at least reflect the home environment where possible. It should, too, relate to where the patient will temporarily spend the major part of his 24-hour day during admission, and also to the staff who will be with him for most of that period (i.e. nursing staff on the ward).

THE MULTIDISCIPLINARY TEAM

The multidisciplinary team is a much-repeated phrase and, when working well, is envied by colleagues who often underestimate the work involved in maintaining it. The difficulties in combining a group of individuals with different backgrounds, attitudes and training who may not be necessarily socially compatible, are huge.

The reason for the team's existence is the patient. This factor is often forgotten, as Fairhurst (1977) reported when 28 case conferences were analysed; more time was spent discussing the work of team members, requests for services, exchange of information and reporting back. Teams come together because they cannot fulfil an objective alone, but team members, as well as the patients they deal with, have needs. Adair (1984) has defined these as task, team maintenance and individual needs (Figure 6.1).

Figure 6.1: Needs of team members (after Adair)

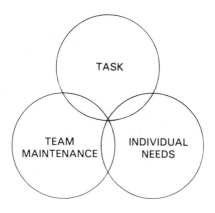

Task needs

This is the reason for the group meeting, and in health care has many levels. At management level it may be determining departmental policy, at case load level it may discuss priorities and routine, and at individual patient/client level the needs of that individual and his immediate carers. At whatever level it exists, of principal importance is the identification and agreement of what the 'task' is.

Team maintenance

The team can be threatened by inside or outside pressures. It may consist of a changing membership, due to rotating staff appointments, and some of its members may be zealous and some burnt-out. Members must be aware of these factors and continually remind themselves of the reason for the team's existence — the patient.

Individual needs

The hierarchy of needs developed by Maslow (1954) is inherent in all of us, and satisfaction of a basic need motivates progress to the next. Individual team members will be at different levels of satisfaction and motivation which can cause difficulties and, again, all members

115

need to be aware of this to ensure understanding of the reaction of others.

The areas of need overlap (Figure 6.1) and can only function as a whole. To this needs to be added the professional and political barriers that unfortunately exist between some professionals for the conclusion to be drawn that teams are not an easy option. Team work is essential to cope with the holistic approach to the older person where no individual can have all the answers.

Effective leadership to co-ordinate the skills of the members is the key to success. This role may be taken by the medical member, but as the doctor does not always play a major role in the patient's rehabilitation, other members may be more appropriate co-ordinators (Richardson 1984).

The report of the Royal Commission on the NHS (1979) identified the following possible difficulties:

(i) The leadership of the team.
(ii) The nature of the corporate responsibility of the team and its effect on the individual members' responsibility.
(iii) Confidentiality.
(iv) Legal aspects of these matters.

The report also acknowledged that the difficulties seen in a multidisciplinary approach are more attributable to inter-professional jealousies than to anything more solid (Brunning and Huffington 1985). These jealousies may result from professional, political or personal reasons and institutions such as hospitals may tend to nurture them. Furnham *et al.* (1981) found that:

(i) Professionals perceive each other negatively if they are in competition over a field of specialisation, a treatment method or a client group.
(ii) Each professional group tends to perceive itself more positively than it perceives another group.

Brunning and Huffington (1985), in drawing attention to the above, describe a workshop where role-playing of a different profession caused participants to support the findings of Furnham, but even after experiencing the problems, participants made no dramatic long-term changes.

Evers (1981) asks several pertinent questions about the team, such as: Who belongs? What are the goals? What is the structure? Who is the leader? How are decisions made? How is work with the patient accomplished? And, what are the care outcomes for the patient? The answers to these questions will vary with each situation, but must be known to team members.

The popularity of the team approach has stood the test of time and must be seen as of value to its participants. It has been suggested (Evers 1981) that helping to cope with uncertainty, support in dealing with a low-status group, and promoting the view that geriatric medicine is uniquely interesting and requires a variety of skills, may support the team concept. Traumatic situations emphasising 'man's inhumanity to man' will also need team support to help professionals deal with their own disgust and frustration (Gibson 1983). Actions such as 'granny bashing', mugging and rape of pensioners are regrettably common items in the media. The Association of Professions for the Mentally Handicapped (APMH) have some useful tips on teamwork which are of value in other settings:

— multiprofessional jargon can be a barrier
— we cannot know everything, but do we know we don't?
— how do others see us, do we hide behind status?
— territorial encroachment needs discussion on the shared areas
— keep personal views separate from ethical debate

(Humphries 1977)

The team should always remember why they are there, and when personal or professional difficulties arise use the patient's problems as the focus for discussion.

The structure of working with a team means that each member will need to give and accept compliments as well as giving and accepting criticism from other members of the team. This can be very hard, especially when people are not used to verbally expressing their feelings in an appropriate way. So each member of the team will need to learn to express their feelings about the patient's concerns and welfare in a manner acceptable to others. Each member of the team will also have to learn to recognise that at different times the main treatment of a certain patient may be in the hands of another member of the team. Trust is important, but so is the ability to challenge decisions and back the challenges with well thought-out observations and reasoning.

Reassessment and review of aims

As already described, goals for the patient are set at the team conference and must be re-evaluated regularly (Henriksen 1978), as changes in physical, mental or social perspectives affect the patient. The collection of information is the task of the whole team (Lefroy 1980) and the data must be shared. The achievement of a plateau, or evidence of deterioration should alert the team to question the relevance of further therapeutic endeavour, or to re-allocate tasks.

Prediction

Prediction of change in the patient's ability and eventual outcome of management is desirable for forward planning, particularly in conjunction with a time-scale.

Elderly people are always difficult to assess and predict because of their capacity for sudden and unexpected change, but attempts have shown themes which all members of the team should consider. Many studies have shown that age need not be a liability in rehabilitation and patients should be seen as individuals with individual problems (De Christopher 1977) but Hodkinson and Hodkinson (1980) found that lower age was a good predictor, and Lamont (1983) found greater age a predictor of deterioration.

Mental status has also been used as a predictor of physical outcome and Hodkinson and Hodkinson (1980) found a higher score a good predictor as did Stewart (1980). Katz (1963) found, and many have since echoed, that dependence in toilet ability was the best indicator dividing subjects into groups receiving significant amounts of assistance.

Predictors should avoid prolonged therapeutic effort in situations where the outcome is unlikely to be successful (Katz 1963); but, when making predictions, Fenwick (1979) warns that we must be clear for whom they are being made, the patient, the family or the bed state.

DISCHARGE

The goal for elderly patients and their carers will normally be discharge to their chosen environment, although a minority of cases will differ because of special circumstances.

If plans are made thoroughly and in good time there can be much satisfaction for the patient, the carers and the team in a job well done, but obstacles to good planning are legion.

Firstly, the patient's readiness for discharge must be established. Discharge for administrative convenience rather than the patient's well-being has been suggested by Evans (1983) as the reason for up to 60 per cent of patients being discharged on a unit's reception day.

Secondly, plans for the discharge must be made and implemented. It is known that a decreased level of independence in some activities occurs after discharge, particularly when equipment is used (Sheikh *et al.* 1979); sufficient time to practise must be allowed. Special requirements, such as wide doorways that have not been met before, also cause loss of independence (Mahoney and Barthel 1965) and time must be allowed for these alterations to be made. The advice of remedial staff should be heeded when discharge is under discussion — Graham and Livesley (1983) found that re-admission occurred earlier when the advice of the remedial staff was disregarded. Re-admission is a daunting prospect for the patient who has 'failed' and to the staff who are implicated in the failure, and to the relative who may feel guilty or exasperated and unwilling to try again. Time spent on planning discharges is time well spent, and communication, again, is the key. Pressure of limited resources will undoubtedly cause regrettable short-cuts to be tried.

EVALUATION

Health care professionals tend to regard record-keeping as time away from the patient, but to progress knowledge and encourage proven effective procedures, evaluation is essential. In its simplest form, checking how many aims were achieved can be recorded (Squires *et al.* 1987). In future, resource allocation may be on the basis of results, as it is in some places already, the facts must replace emotion in the evaluation of our intervention, what the result is, duration, quantity and effect. This applies to all disciplines and numerous team-recording procedures have been described (Israel *et al.* 1984).

WARD FACILITIES

For rehabilitation to be a 24-hour process it is vital that the patient's environment is suited to his need and changes as his needs do. All too often the first chair the patient sits on becomes 'his' whether suitable or not. The distance to the toilet, availability of walking aids (hopefully not stored neatly in the corner) named for the owner, variety in height and positions of aids in the toilet, should be considered in the context of the whole ward. Dignity encourages rehabilitation and teeth, hearing aids, glasses, clothing and shoes should all be provided and accessible for the patient on an individual basis.

It is easy for staff to become institutionalised in their own institution and fail to notice what they would observe elsewhere with horror.

SUMMARY

Identification of the patient's potential for rehabilitation or not is an essential first step. Members of the multidisciplinary team will all have contributions to make and receive and this effective functioning of the team is the key to good geriatric care. The patient and his carer should be regarded as part of the team and listened to and informed at all stages. Realistic intervention must be monitored for effectiveness and aims altered in the light of results. Discharge should be well planned for maximum success.

Patients who, because of their frailty and prognosis, may be appropriate to receive tender loving care rather than rehabilitation, should still be regarded as people with needs, as should their carers. Death at the end of a full life can still be seen positively, but inexperienced relatives and staff may need help to cope.

As can be seen the term 'rehabilitation' is a wide and complex subject. Experience is gained with each patient and team contact and communication is the key. It has been said that 'one could argue for greater expertise with greater age' (Hunter 1986).

REFERENCES

Adair, J. (1984) *The Skills of Leadership*. Gower, London

Brunning, H. and Huffington, C. (1985) Altered image. *Nursing Times*, 31 July

Coates, H. and King, A. (1982) *The Patient Assessment*. Churchill Livingstone, Edinburgh

De Christopher, J. (1977) Factors important in geriatric rehabilitation; need age be a liability? *American Research Nursing Journal*, 2, 4, 9–17

Denham, M. (ed.) (1983) *Care of the Long Stay Elderly Patient*. Croom Helm, London

Evans, J.G. (1983) The appraisal of hospital geriatric services. *Community Medicine*, 5, 242–50

Evers, H. (1981) Multidisciplinary teams in geriatric wards: Myth or reality? *Journal of Advanced Nursing*, 6, 205–14

Fairhurst, E. (1977) Teamwork as panacea: some underlying assumptions. Unpublished paper read at the annual congress of the Medical Sociology Group of the British Sociological Association

Fenwick, A. (1979) An interdisciplinary tool for assessing patients' readiness for discharge in the rehabilitation setting. *Journal of Advanced Nursing*, 4, 9–21

Furnham, A., Pendleton, D. and Mannicom, C. (1981) The perception of different occupations within the medical professions. *Social Science and Medicine*, 15E, 289–300

Gibson, M. (1983) Teamwork in caring. *Contact Pastoral Care Magazine*, 13–16

Graham, H. and Livesley, B. (1983) Can re-admission to a geriatric medical unit be prevented? *Lancet*, 1 (8321), 404–6

Grant, E. (1985) Survey of the use of aids to daily living by physically handicapped people. In *Manpower Services Commission project*, School of Bio-Medical Engineering, University of Dundee, Scotland

Guidex, C. (1986) Quality vs quantity? *Centre for Health Economics Newsletter*, 1, York

Henriksen, J.D. (1978) Problems in rehabilitation after age sixty-five. *Journal of the American Geriatrics Society*, 26, 11, 510–12

Hesse, K. and Campion, E. (1983) Motivating the geriatric patient for rehabilitation. *Journal of the American Geriatrics Society*, 31, 10, 586–9

Hodkinson, H. and Hodkinson, I. (1980) The influence of route of admission on outcome in the geriatric patient. *Age and Ageing*, 9, 229–34

Humphries, K. (1977) *Working Together — Aspects of Providing a Multidisciplinary Service for Mentally Handicapped People*. Association of Professions for the Mentally Handicapped, London

Hunter, A. (1986) A positive attitude to priority services. *Therapy Weekly*, 12, 4

Isaacs, B. (1986) Ultimately Immobile patients in departments of geriatric medicine. *Journal of the Royal Society of Health*, 2, 49–50

Israel, L., Kozarevic, D. and Sartorius, N. (1984) *The Source Book of Geriatric Assessments*. Karger, New York

Katz, S. (1963) Studies of illness in the aged. *Journal of the American Medical Association*, 185, 12, 914–19

Lamont, C. (1983) The outcome of hospitalisation for acute illness in the elderly. *Journal of the American Geriatrics Society*, 31, 5, 282–8

Lefroy, R.B. (1980) Assessment of disabilities. *Medical Journal of Australia, 1,* 635–6

Mahoney, F. and Barthel, D.W. (1965) Functional evaluation: the Barthel Index. *Maryland State Medical Journal, 14,* 61–5

Maslow, A.H. (1954) *Motivation & Personality.* Harper, New York

Mort, M. (1985) *Retraining for the Elderly Disabled.* Croom Helm, London

Nicholls, P.R.J. (1976) Are ADL indices of any value? *British Journal of Occupational Therapists, 6,* 160–3

Ransome, H. (1978) Rehabilitation principles applied to physiotherapy for the elderly. In V. Carver and P. Liddiard (eds), *An Ageing Population.* Hodder & Stoughton, London

Reed, J. and Gessner, J. (1979) Rehabilitation in the extended care facility. *Journal of the American Geriatrics Society, 27,* 7, 325–9

Richardson, B. (1984) Rehabilitation in a multidisciplinary setting. *New Zealand Journal of Physiotherapy, 4,* 35–6

Rosenberg, W., Parkes, J., Jenkins, A., Denham, M., Royston, J., Sullens, C., O'Neill, C. and Dobbs, S. (1986) Making a rehabilitation hospital for the elderly work. *Health Trends, 18,* 3, 66–71

Royal Commission on the NHS (1979) Report. HMSO, London

Rubenstein, I., Schaver, C., Weland, G. and Kane, R. (1984) Systematic bias in functional assessment of elderly adults; effects of different data sources. *Journal of Gerontology, 39,* 6, 686–91

Sheikh, K., Smith, D., Meade, T., Goldenberg, E., Brennan, P. and Kinsella, G. (1979) Repeatability and validity of a modified ADL index in studies of chronic disability. *International Rehabilitation Medicine, 1,* 51–8

Squires, A., Dolbear, R., Williams, R. and Smoker, S. (1987) Evaluation of physiotherapy in a day unit. *Physiotherapy, 73,* 11, 596–8

Stewart, C.P.U. (1980) A prediction score for geriatric rehabilitation prospects. *Rheumatology and Rehabilitation, 19,* 239–45

Stokes-Roberts, A. (1986) Maintaining activities and interests. In S. Redfern (ed.), *Nursing Elderly People.* Churchill Livingstone, Edinburgh

Suchett-Kaye, A., Sarker, U., Elkan, G. and Waring, M. (1971) Physical, mental and social assessments of patients suffering from CVA with special reference to rehabilitation. *Gerontology Clinica, 13,* 192–206

7

The Role of the Nurse in Rehabilitation

Linda Thomas

INTRODUCTION

The concept of a multidisciplinary team in which several health-care professionals work together as equals for the good of the patient is excellent. However, no team can work effectively unless each member clearly understands the role of every other member.

In terms of health care, one of the greatest difficulties in creating a successful multidisciplinary team approach tends to be that each discipline thinks it understands exactly what all the other disciplines do. Nurses suffer particularly from stereotyping, including the much beloved 'angel' image promulgated by romantic works of fiction and the tabloid press.

Thus the foundations are laid for interpretation of the role of the nurse as a 'doer' and the (doctor's) patient as the 'done to'. In fact, the art of geriatric nursing has been defined as the enlightened withdrawal of nursing support (Coni *et al.* 1980). However, when viewed from a historical perspective, it can be seen that this definition is a relatively new interpretation of the role of the nurse in the care of elderly people. The developing role of the hospital nurse in the United Kingdom will be examined here.

REHABILITATION OF ELDERLY PEOPLE

A historical nursing perspective

The institutional care of elderly people is rooted in the Poor Law Acts, most notably the Poor Law Amendment Act of 1834. It was intended that this Act would ensure that relief available to able-bodied paupers within the workhouse would never be greater than any relief which was available outside. Workhouses were therefore suitably grim and prisonlike.

The needs of elderly people were not considered separately from those of the poor in general, and for those elderly inmates who were unfortunate enough to need care in the workhouse infirmary, contemporary accounts of the conditions are graphic. Care was provided by 'nurses' who were in fact workhouse paupers themselves.

> . . . the general character of the nursing will be appreciated by the details of the one fact, that we found in one ward two paralytic patients with frightful sloughs of the back; they were both dirty and lying on hard straw mattresses — the one dressed only with a rag steeped in chloride of lime solution, the other with a rag thickly covered with ointment. The latter was a fearful and very extensive sore, in a state of absolute putridity: the buttocks of the patient were covered with filth and excoriated and the stench was masked by strewing dry chloride of lime on the floor under the bed. A spectacle more saddening and more discreditable cannot be imagined.

Dean and Bolton (1980) quote this example from 'The *Lancet* Sanitary Commission for Investigation into the State of the Infirmaries of Workhouses' from the *Lancet*, 12 August 1865, noting that it exemplifies growing demands for workhouse reform at that time.

Medical and nursing developments

Nevertheless, nearly a century later in the 1930s custodial care was still the order of the day when Dr Marjory Warren of the West Middlesex Hospital assumed responsibility for more than 800 people in the chronic wards of a former workhouse infirmary. Dr Warren became the first medical practitioner to recognise that elderly people should have the same right of access to assessment, diagnostic and therapeutic facilities as any other age group.

This policy of active treatment for elderly patients who had previously been condemned to a life in bed meant that, by 1948, Dr Warren had succeeded in reducing the number of beds in the chronic wards to 200. Regrettably, as with many pioneers, Dr Warren lacked the wholehearted support of her medical colleagues and it was to be many years before her philosophy of care was widely adopted.

A booklet written by Dr Warren (undated, probably early 1950s) on the treatment and care of elderly patients drew attention to the need for pioneering work to be undertaken by nurses in places where elderly people were being treated by out-of-date methods. Due to the efforts of a nurse named Doreen Norton who had read and been inspired by the booklet, by 1959 a geriatric nursing research unit had been established at the Whittington Hospital in London. In collaboration with colleagues, Doreen Norton began research which culminated in *An Investigation of Geriatric Nursing Problems in Hospital* (Norton *et al.* 1962).

Norton has subsequently described vividly (1986) the type of care being given to elderly patients in hospital throughout this period:

> Picture the scene: a big open ward with dark brown or bottle green paintwork and a forest of cotbeds at one end; at least two thirds of its inhabitants bedfast, grossly incontinent and, for the most part, reliving in mind and deed episodes in a life long gone. No physiotherapist ever trod its shiny floor but an occupational therapist came occasionally to supply the few more alert ladies with knitting — usually huge knitting needles and a ball of twine for making dishcloths; the men did nothing much, except smoke their pipes and leave ash all over the bed. Death was usually the only form of discharge, for attitudes were such that an old person's place in the community vanished automatically with admission.

It is very difficult to track down the moment at which it was decided, during the 1950s, that nursing elderly people in bed permanently might be harmful to them. By all accounts, it seems to have been almost an overnight decision and the end result of this 'progress' in care suggests that previously bedfast patients simply became chairbound instead.

The wards, of course, were hopelessly ill-equipped for this development in care. There had never been the need before for sitting rooms, or roomy bathrooms to cater for heavily dependent patients, or hoists, or numerous commodes, or variable height beds, or walking aids, or any of the other paraphernalia of rehabilitation. The needs of a bedbound patient are very simple. Modern approaches to geriatric care are still frequently accommodated in these old buildings with their architectural inadequacies — often part of the main structure and difficult and expensive to alter.

REVOLUTION IN CARE

Throughout the 1960s, an increasing number of articles and reports appeared reflecting both developments and problems in geriatric care. Few were written by nurses, although many had implications for nursing. For example, Denham (1983) has drawn attention to many articles of this period which recognised the dehumanising effect on elderly people of the regimented system of care.

Then in 1967 came the shocking revelations published in *Sans Everything* (Robb 1967), a collection of eye-witness reports from nurses and others which highlighted incidents of cruelty, neglect and inhumane treatment of elderly people in both general and psychiatric hospitals.

Against this chequered background, it becomes easier to understand just how far the nursing care of elderly people has progressed to achieve its current status as a speciality. Nevertheless, it is also worth remembering that the revolution is a recent one. It is inevitable that in some areas, the ethos of custodial care may linger on. Nurses trained in the 'traditional' ways of nursing in the 1950s and 1960s may sometimes have experienced difficulties in adapting to a rapidly evolving speciality where the promotion of independence for the elderly patient is paramount.

Many factors have contributed to this apparent unwillingness to accept the change in philosophy; lack of imaginative support from managers, limited or non-existent access to post-basic and in-service training programmes, inadequate and overcrowded facilities, poor staffing levels and recruitment difficulties are some of the most common problems leading to low morale and lack of motivation.

Fortunately, this type of situation is becoming much less common and the growth of interest in the speciality has been reflected in developments within nurse education. Since 1979, it has become a statutory requirement of nurse training in the United Kingdom that all learner nurses must undertake practical experience in the specialised care of elderly people during their training.

Furthermore, there are now post-basic courses available for qualified nurses who wish to further their knowledge, as outlined below.

THE NURSE AS MEMBER OF A TEAM

It is questionable whether nurses have ever been accorded equal status with other members of the multidisciplinary team. This may be due, in part, to the old-fashioned stereotyped image of the nurse as the doctor's 'handmaiden'. Nevertheless, nursing itself must share part of the blame in what has been perceived as its inability to define the nursing role.

This too is changing; the introduction of the Nursing Process in the late 1970s and early 1980s provided the opportunity for developing a logical and systematic method of planning packages of nursing care tailored to meet the needs of individual patients. This move away from 'task allocation' towards patient-centred nursing care has been widely accepted as the most effective means of organising and delivering care (Royal College of Nursing 1981).

Most importantly, the nursing process allows for information about patients — which had previously been locked safely and inaccessibly within the brain of the nurse in charge — to be written down and thereby shared, not only with other nurses, but also with the rest of the team.

The concept of shared interdisciplinary care plans is now being discussed in progressive units specialising in the care of elderly people, an idea made ever more feasible by the increasing interest in computer technology and its possible application to patient care planning. (See also Chapter 14.)

In those areas where the implementation of individualised patient care planning has been introduced with proper preparation, nursing care of patients has improved noticeably (Miller 1985). Another recent development which is likely to make a considerable impact on changing nursing practice, particularly in relation to rehabilitation, is the notion of nursing models. Several different models have been described; an outline of the philosophies of two of the most commonly used models is found below.

EXAMPLES OF NURSING MODELS

Orem's self-care model for nursing

Developed by Dorothea Orem (1980), the three parts of this model are:

(i) Universal self-care requisites (basic human needs such as food, water, air, etc.).

(ii) Developmental self-care requisites (related, for example, to life changes — perhaps bereavement or unemployment).

(iii) Health deviation self-care requisites (where the individual's ability for self-care is affected by ill-health).

The overriding goal of this model has been described by Pearson and Vaughan (1986) as the elimination of self-care deficits.

Roper's activities of living model for nursing

Developed by Nancy Roper, Winifred Logan and Alison Tierney (1981), this model describes twelve basic activities of living — for example: maintaining a safe environment, breathing, eliminating, sleeping — some of which may be affected by the individual's stage in the lifespan (expressing sexuality would be inapplicable to babies). In applying a problem-solving approach to this model, nurses also need to know the physical, sociological and psychological aspects of the twelve identified activities of living.

CONTINUITY OF NURSING CARE

In hospital

When patients are admitted to hospital, they can confidently expect that a nursing service will be provided 24 hours of the day, every day of the year. This continuity of care has obvious implications for nurses as members of the team in that they are usually in the best position to note changes in a patient's condition. This may be of particular significance if, for example, a patient who is progressing well towards discharge home and functioning more or less independently throughout the day becomes regularly confused with episodes of incontinence at night. A review of night-time medication by medical staff may solve the problem provided the night nursing staff are properly involved as members of the team.

Nurses are also more likely to come into contact at a very early stage with a patient's relatives or other informal carers and are often able to identify significant problems which may occur in the home

Figure 7.1: Nurses' discharge checklist

PATIENT	YES	NO	DATE	COMMENTS SIGNATURE
Patient informed				
Relatives/carers informed				
Transport arranged				
Access to home confirmed/keys available				
Property/valuables returned				
MEDICATION: Ordered Given to patient with explanation				
Home help				
Meals on wheels				
Community nurse				
Health visitor				
Community psychiatric nurse				
Outpatient department appointment				
Day Hospital appointment				
Discharge letter to GP				

situation long before a home visit is arranged to assess the patient's ability to cope. While the doctor may well be perceived as the team leader, it is generally nurses who find themselves in the role of team coordinators.

This is perhaps best illustrated by the example of a discharge planning checklist. Discharging an elderly patient from hospital can be a complex undertaking which involves a tremendous amount of advance planning and the imparting of information to a wide variety of different people, both lay and professional. As Figure 7.1 shows, it is invariably the nurse who has the most involvement in co-ordinating these arrangements.

Given all these factors, it is obviously vitally important that nurses are fully involved in ward rounds and case conferences and that their views and opinions are sought and respected in planning rehabilitation and treatment programmes. Otherwise situations are likely to arise where, for example, a patient who has been painstakingly helped to walk with minimal assistance in the physiotherapy department all week is taken everywhere in a wheelchair by nurses all weekend.

Community liaison

Many units specialising in the care of elderly people have community-liaison nurses attached to them, usually either district nurses or health visitors, part of whose role is to ease communication between hospital and community staff. Most community-liaison nurses attend ward rounds and case conferences and offer follow-up visits to patients following discharge. However, there has been little evaluation of the effectiveness of these posts (Ross 1986).

In the community

The Council for the Education and Training of Health Visitors (CETHV) defined the functions of the health visitor as follows:

— prevention of mental, physical and emotional ill-health or alleviation of its consequences
— early detection of ill-health and the surveillance of high-risk groups
— recognition and identification of need, and mobilisation of resources where necessary
— provision of care; this will include support during periods of stress, and advice and guidance in case of illness (CETHV 1977).

Unfortunately, it is generally recognised that the skills of health visitors are by no means utilised to the full in the care of elderly people. Although there are some who have chosen to specialise in the care of this client group, in reality very few health visitors have much contact with elderly people (While 1986).

By contrast, district nurses spend virtually three-quarters of their time caring for elderly people (Dunnell and Dobbs 1982). District nurses may have either a geographical responsibility or they may be general practitioner 'attached'. While the organisational concepts may differ, the system of delivering nursing care is the same in that it is generally based on the nursing process approach.

Since 1981, it has become mandatory for district nurses to undertake a nine-month training course based at institutes of higher education and including three months supervised practice. The district nurse may then lead a nursing team which comprises registered nurses (those who have not undertaken the mandatory training), enrolled nurses (who, following a two-year basic training as opposed to the three-year training of the registered nurse, may or may not have undertaken the mandatory training) and nursing auxiliaries.

The role of the district nurse with elderly people varies widely according to the needs of each individual client. District nurses may offer advice on lifting skills and the prevention of pressure sores to informal carers of dependants at home; as part of a team, they may help in devising rehabilitation programmes, for example for patients who have suffered strokes (and who may not have been hospitalised at all). They may become involved in promoting continence or managing incontinence effectively, administering drugs and monitoring compliance, providing nursing aids and so on. The Department of Health and Social Security (1981) discovered that district nurses spend 27 per cent of their time looking after patients over the age of 65 who have leg ulcers.

Taking into account the complex nature of the district nurse's role, the suggestion that a shared professional record kept in the home at the point of delivery of care in order to promote coordination and prevent fragmentation of professional resources especially for housebound elderly people seems an excellent idea (Ross 1986).

As well as district nurses and health visitors, the move away from institutional care to care in the community in the past few years has led to a great increase in the numbers of community psychiatric nurses and community nurses caring for clients with a mental handicap. It is also worth bearing in mind that a growing number of nurses have chosen to specialise in different areas of care with very specific interests. They often have both hospital and community responsibilities and can be invaluable resources to all members of the team in planning rehabilitation programmes — the continence advisor is one good example.

ROLE OF THE CONTINENCE ADVISOR

The Association of Continence Advisors (1985) has defined the primary function of the continence advisor as that of promoting continence by providing an educational/advisory service for professional and others caring for the incontinent person. Continence advisors may be either hospital- or community-based nurses and may work alone or as part of a team, for example in a urodynamics clinic. The principal areas covered tend to be:

Clinical

Perhaps with a small case load, both in hospital and the community. Involvement with other professionals in continence advisory clinics.

Educational

Informal and formal teaching of all those involved in caring for incontinent people on the promotion of continence and the management of incontinence, including health and social services staff, voluntary organisations and the general public, etc.

Liaison

With supplies and linen services managers, commercial organisations, health education officers, finance officers, as well as all members of the multidisciplinary team.

Research

On all aspects of the promotion of continence and the management of incontinence, including the evaluation of equipment.

Advisory

Most continence advisors, particularly if they have a regional responsibility, offer an information and resource service.

UNDERSTANDING NURSING PROBLEMS

Even the most enthusiastic nurses may occasionally be disheartened in their attempts to plan and implement rehabilitation programmes for their patients. There are numerous problems which occur to thwart the best-laid plans, some of which are easily solved when communications are improved with the rest of the team, and some of which are rather more complex.

Cultural

The phrase 'being cruel to be kind' is one often heard in connection with the rehabilitation of elderly people and it perhaps epitomises one of the most profound conflicts of nursing, as discussed by Norman (1980): the desire to protect patients weighed against the desire to promote independence and allow patients to take risks.

The whole ethos of nursing care tends to be directed towards protecting the patient from harm. Cultural influences may foster an attitude of promoting dependence in a patient rather than independence; indeed, Miller (1985) has identified that traditional nursing is associated with increased patient dependency. Taken to the extreme, the protective instinct may involve the use of restraints such as cotsides or tipped back 'geriatric' chairs with lockable table fronts. The latter, used without team consultation, can lead to much disagreement as balance can be affected, in addition to incontinence, frustration and anxiety being caused. In a few cases these chairs *may* be the only answer — but with the variety of seating now available a better alternative should be sought by the team.

In allowing patients to take the risks inevitable and inherent in an active atmosphere of rehabilitation, much depends on the willingness of managers to understand this philosophy of care and to recognise that blame should not be unfairly apportioned. Other members of the team can always play a supportive role in helping to educate the uninitiated.

Circumstantial

In 1975, the Joint Working Party of the Nursing and Remedial Professions published a report, *Health Services Management*, which made reference to 'intrinsic overlap' where certain skills are shared by more than one profession, and 'circumstantial overlap' where members of one profession undertake something which is not part of their normal role because a member of the appropriate profession is not available.

Despite the fact that shortages of nursing staff remain a constant problem both in the community and on most wards caring for elderly people in United Kingdom hospitals, the difficulties arising from circumstantial overlap have never really been addressed. The advice of the 1975 Working Party (whose report appeared as a Health Circular), that a pattern of work should be discussed and agreed between the professions concerned, including the provision of therapist advice to nurses working on different shifts, still holds good.

Environmental

There are now many attractive and well-designed hospital units specialising in the care of elderly people; upgrading programmes have become ever more imaginative and sensitive to the needs of elderly people and the staff caring for them. The Health Building Note produced by the Welsh Office of the DHSS (1981) on hospital accommodation for elderly people is full of sound advice and guidance for those concerned with the provision and design of new health buildings and the adaptation or extension of existing premises.

Unfortunately, however, poorly designed and overcrowded wards and hospitals remain a fact of life in too many places. Wells (1980) stressed the need for administrators to relate their plans directly to actual patient care, always having on all planning committees informed, vocal ward sisters/charge nurses. One simple example of how environmental influences directly affect the nursing care and rehabilitation of patients is in the provision of toilets. Planning a continence training programme may be virtually impossible if toilets are scarce and distant from the day area or bed area. Similarly, the toilet space may not allow for manoeuvring a wheelchair, and there may not be enough space in the ward to allow for a commode to be left by the bed at night.

Nurses caring for elderly people in the community will also experience problems relating to the environment. Age Concern (1980) has pointed out that elderly people are more likely than younger ones to live in houses built before 1919; and also to live in privately rented accommodation and, therefore, to be without certain basic amenities such as an indoor toilet or fixed hot bath or shower. Unsuitable accommodation may affect the activity levels of elderly people at home; for the housebound minority of the over-75s there is also an increased risk of falling (Thomas 1985).

Elderly people at home may have difficulty in negotiating stairs and steps; door widths may prevent wheelchairs from being used around the house; Rollator frames may be unusable on carpets. Lack of space generally may make it difficult to use hoists or commodes or other basic equipment. All these are factors which need to be taken into account by district nurses and health visitors.

Equipment

The frustration engendered by inappropriate or poorly maintained equipment can be just as great as that caused by lack of space. Nothing is more irritating than a wheelchair with flat tyres and footrests missing and no planned programme for maintenance.

Most hospital wards now have variable height beds, but nurses in the community may need to exercise considerable ingenuity in caring for an elderly and perhaps incontinent patient in a vast double bed in a tiny bedroom.

Unfortunately, nurses are not always aware of the wide range of chair designs which support the concept of chairs as 'therapeutic tools' (Wells 1980). The idea that a chair is a chair is a chair is often reinforced when, for example, a brand new unit is opened equipped with armchairs which are all identical in every detail, chosen to match the decor of the new ward and not to match the individual patient's needs.

The multiplicity of problems associated with the lack of adequate provision of personalised clothing systems is another area which directly affects nursing care. A patient is hardly likely to feel very enthusiastic about attempting to mobilise if her dress does not fit, or his trousers have no belt or braces and are liable to fall down or if stockings are precariously (and perhaps painfully) kept up by knots above the knee, or if a split-back dress is likely to fly open to reveal that no knickers have been supplied. Footwear can be equally hazardous. There are very few units which can honestly claim to be providing a decent and dignified standard of supply and/or laundering.

Staffing levels

All of these problems may be compounded by inadequate staffing levels or an inappropriate mix of staff so that there are insufficient trained nursing staff to monitor and supervise the work of learner nurses and nursing auxiliaries.

Today, there are suggestions and recommendations as to how nurse education in the United Kingdom should be reformed for all specialities (Project 2000 1986).

WORKING TOGETHER

The multidisciplinary team may vary in size and membership but it is essential that all members of the team work together and communicate effectively if the best interests of the patient are to be kept at heart. Developing a joint strategy in planning a patient's rehabilitation programme becomes something of a nonsense if, for example, the patient is hurriedly dressed by nurses on the ward because occupational therapists insist that the patient must be in their department by 9.30 a.m. — for dressing practice!

Once this type of fundamental breakdown of communication is addressed and put right, members of the team can begin to develop joint approaches to planning care. Serious consideration must be given to the possibility of promoting the use of joint written care plans and, in the meantime, nursing care plan documentation can be enormously helpful as a means of communication.

It is extraordinarily difficult to rehabilitate an elderly person realistically without some idea of the home circumstances to which he or she is returning. Home visits are obviously very helpful, but the involvement of the district nurse or health visitor at an early stage may throw some light on problems which might otherwise not be identified. Ideally, community staff should be informed of and present during home visits.

The expertise of all members of the team should be sought and acted upon when upgrading is planned or new building programmes commissioned, and when new equipment such as chairs or hoists are to be purchased. Sometimes, failure to involve each other in this type of decision is by no means deliberate but simply due to thoughtlessness; making a conscious effort to think about who should be consulted is a step in the right direction to working together effectively.

SUMMARY

There is more to nursing than making beds and giving out bedpans, more to occupational therapy than dishing out knitting needles, more to physiotherapy than muscle development, more to chiropody than cutting toenails — and more to being part of a multidisciplinary team than attending ward rounds and case conferences.

Each member of the team has a responsibility to communicate with other members of the team with respect as equals. Sometimes a member of the team may expose a lack of knowledge or make a mistake and then it is all too easy to criticise or patronise when a little sympathy or tactful education might be far more constructive.

Building professional barriers is not at all difficult; breaking down the barriers which have already been built is hard work, but worth it in the end. The rewards of seeing a patient fulfil his or her maximum potential and knowing that it is a result of good teamwork are enormous.

REFERENCES

Age Concern (1980) *Profiles of the Elderly: Their Housing*. Age Concern, Mitcham, Research Publication 5:7

Association of Continence Advisors (1985) *Guidelines on the Role of the District Continence Advisor*. Association of Continence Advisors, London

Coni, N., Davidson, W. and Webster, S. (1980) *Lecture Notes on Geriatrics*. Blackwell Scientific Publications, Oxford, 2nd edn

Council for the Education and Training of Health Visitors (1977) *An Investigation into the Principles of Health Visiting*. CETHV, London

Dean, M. and Bolton, G. (1980) The Administration of Poverty. In C. Davies (ed.) *Rewriting Nursing History*. Croom Helm, London

Denham, M.J. (ed.) (1983) *Care of the Long-Stay Elderly Patient*. Croom Helm, London

Department of Health and Social Security (1981) *Report of a Study on Community Care*. HMSO, London

———— (Welsh Office) (1981) Hospital Accommodation for Elderly People. In *Health Building Note 37*, HMSO, London

Dunnell, K. and Dobbs, J. (1982) *Nurses Working in the Community*. Office of Population Censuses and Surveys, London

Health Services Management (1975) Report of the Joint Working Party of the Nursing and Remedial Professions. Health Circular (77)124 DHSS, London

Miller, A. (1985) Does the process help the patient? *Nursing Times*, 26 June

Norman, A.J. (1980) *Rights and Risk: a discussion document on civil liberty in old age*. National Council for the Care of Old People (now Centre for Policy on Ageing), London

Norton, D., McCaren, R. and Exton-Smith, A.N. (1962) *An Investigation of Geriatric Nursing Problems in Hospital*. National Corporation for the Care of Old People. (Reprinted 1976, Churchill Livingstone, Edinburgh.)

Norton, D. (1986) The Past is the Key to the Future. Unpublished paper given at the Royal College of Nursing Society of Geriatric Nursing Conference, Nottingham, 10 September

Orem, D. (1980) *Nursing — Concepts of Practice*. McGraw Hill, New York, 2nd edn

Pearson, A. and Vaughan, B. (1986) *Nursing Models for Practice*. Heinemann, London

Project 2000; A New Preparation for Practice. (1986) United Kingdom Central Council, London

Robb, B. (1967) *Sans Everything — A Case to Answer*. Aegis Publication, Thomas Nelson, London

Roper, N., Logan, W. and Tierney, A. (1981) *Learning to Use the Process of Nursing*. Churchill Livingstone, Edinburgh

Ross, F.M. (1986) Nursing Old People in the Community. In S. Redfern (ed.) *Nursing Elderly People*. Churchill Livingstone, Edinburgh

Royal College of Nursing (1981) *Towards Standards — A Discussion Document*. Royal College of Nursing, London

Thomas, L. (1985) *Learning to Care for Elderly People*. Hodder and Stoughton, Sevenoaks

Warren, M. (undated) Treatment and Care of Elderly Patients. Booklet reprinted from the *Hospital and Social Service Journal*

Wells, T.J. (1980) *Problems in Geriatric Nursing Care*. Churchill Livingstone, Edinburgh

While, A.E. (1986) Health Visiting and the Elderly. In S. Redfern (ed.) *Nursing Elderly People*. Churchill Livingstone, Edinburgh

8

Feet and Footwear of Older People

Judith Kemp

INTRODUCTION

An important part of rehabilitation for most older people is the renewal of their ability to move about independently. Whilst relatively few are faced with being wheelchair bound, many find difficulty in walking following major episodes of ill-health, particularly if their illness has affected muscle power or control, the circulation or the innervation of the lower limb. Prolonged bed rest is now rare post-operatively, but loss of muscle power is rapid in onset in older people. The importance of early mobilisation and/or intensive physiotherapy to maintain or restore muscle power cannot be over-emphasised.

However, if the patient has painful feet or inadequate footwear they will inevitably be reluctant or incapable of walking about, especially if this is coupled with an already low morale or motivation.

Painful feet amongst the elderly population are by no means rare. Many elderly people manage to live with their foot problems for years, but an episode of ill-health can make the need for chiropody treatment become apparent. Of people aged 65 and over, recent surveys (Clarke 1969; Kemp and Winkler 1983; Cartwright and Henderson 1987) show that between 50 and 80 per cent of elderly people have some sort of foot problem. Some of these will be relatively minor in themselves, such as thickened or distorted nails or corns and callouses. It is when these are found in conjunction with general frailty or systemic disorders such as rheumatoid arthritis or diabetes mellitus that there is the potential for severe disability. Even when the feet show no abnormality the patient may

139

be in pain from over-long toenails which they cannot cut due to poor grip, stiff spine or hips, or following surgery such as hip replacement. Whilst relatives may perform this simple task, it is not usually the sort of thing one could ask a neighbour to do.

Foot deformities such as hallux valgus (bunion) will lead to a reduction in the efficiency of foot function, severe difficulty in finding or wearing 'normal' footwear, and increased tendency to foot lesions including ulceration.

Abnormal foot function is probably the commonest cause of foot deformity, and many of the foot problems presented by older patients are symptoms of this abnormal functioning.

In many cases, minor abnormalities, inherited at birth or acquired in childhood have gone unnoticed until middle or old age. School medical services were in their infancy when today's elderly people were eligible for school foot inspections. By this time, compensatory changes will have taken place in the joint surfaces making correction impossible. Accompanying soft tissue changes will also have occurred and some correction of these may be possible to improve function. Abnormalities of function detected in children can sometimes be corrected permanently, and can frequently be controlled in adults, lessening the secondary effects by the use of functional orthoses. These stabilise the rear foot or correct movement (usually at the sub talar and mid tarsal joints) producing a more normal foot function without producing anatomical correction.

Having laid emphasis on the mechanical function of the foot, it must not be forgotten that foot problems also include infections, and lesions of the skin and nails. It is usually these which bring the feet to notice, as few patients will present asking for treatment of their foot function. In addition, the normal ageing process can affect mobility and many systemic disorders have consequences for the foot and lower limb.

THE CHIROPODIAL APPROACH TO FOOT PROBLEMS

As with all rehabilitative procedures, the approach to foot problems will include diagnosis, assessment and prognosis, and treatment. The processes of these will now be discussed.

Diagnosis

This must include both diagnosis of the foot problems and the knowledge of the diagnoses of any other medical, surgical and psychiatric conditions, all of which may affect the feet. Likewise, particular drug therapies may affect the tissues of the feet. Surgery, especially to the hip or lower limb will also be particularly relevant.

Structural and functional deformity A brief bio-mechanical examination will give the chiropodist information about the stability and mobility of the foot. The relationship between calcaneum and lower leg (with the sub talar joint in neutral) can be determined. This is important as if the calcaneum is inverted or everted to the leg, there will probably be deformities in the forefoot. It is important to detect the cause of forefoot deformities, as treatment may also need to be directed at the rearfoot problem. Examination of the sub talar, mid tarsal and tarso-metatarsal joint motions will further reveal abnormalities of the relationship between the rearfoot and forefoot.

The range of motion at other joints will also be tested, both passively and by the patient performing active movements. Observation of gait will include scanning of head, shoulder level, arm swing, spinal alignment, hip level and the relationship of the knees to detect problems which may contribute to, cause, or result from foot problems.

Finally, the chiropodist may examine the footwear if available, as the distortion of the uppers, and the wear marks on the soles can give useful information about gait.

Skin and soft tissue examination An examination of the skin will reveal skin lesions which may range from minor callousities, through to major problems such as skin cancers. The colour and temperature of the skin give indications of the circulation. The posterior tibial and dorsalis pedis pulses will be palpated, and many chiropodists now use doppler ultrasound for examining the circulation in the lower limb. Sensation tests for vibration, temperature and light touch will also be performed. Signs of systemic skin disease and infections will be noted. Conditions of deeper tissues, including bursitis, tenosynovitis and heel pain will also be recorded.

Toenails will be examined for distorted growth or infections. Infected lesions of nails or skin will be swabbed for identification of the causative agents prior to commencement of treatment.

Assessment and prognosis

The chiropodist will next assess the potential for treatment success, as the co-operation of the patient will be very important in particular types of treatment. Some problems, such as long or deformed toenails are instantly relieved by treatment, whilst others such as ulcers may be slower to respond. Structural deformities may be impossible to cure, but the associated problems such as bursitis or corns will be helped by chiropodial treatment. In such cases immediate treatment will help, although long-term treatment has to be planned, usually including a change of footwear.

Assessment of any given treatment's suitability will be modified by the patient's general health. Thus radical treatments may be rejected because of underlying systemic disease. The chiropodist will produce a treatment plan, including a prognosis, taking into account all relevant factors.

Treatment

As indicated already, there are differing time-scales in which treatment can be effective. These are:

— short-term treatment to relieve immediate problems
— medium-term treatment using adhesive padding to predict the likely outcome of long-term treatment
— long-term treatment with permanent orthoses, other appliances or shoe adaptations

The object of all three stages is to bring the feet to the optimum state possible, and to maximise foot function. Whilst treatment can be divided by time-scale, it is probably more useful to divide this discussion of foot problems by the structures affected.

Skeletal deformities Skeletal deformities can be divided into whole foot deformities and those affecting either the rearfoot or forefoot.

Whole foot deformities include pes cavus and pes planus, and all the talipes deformities. Many of these will have been present from birth, and in old age will usually present as a rigid foot. Each deformity will bring its own characteristic lesions but the principles of treatment will include debridement of callous and removal of corns, the use of protective padding, and provision of insoles to increase weight-bearing where necessary, and relieve overloaded areas. Provision of specialised footwear will be essential, although many of these patients will have such shoes already.

Ankle equinus can be acquired, due to long years of wearing high heels, as the tendo achilles group of muscles gradually shorten. It is not advisable for the patient to go into flat shoes, but to wear the lowest heels which give comfort. The heels should be chunky to improve stability.

Rearfoot deformities in older people may be the result of untreated congenital problems such as osseus bars between the bones of the rearfoot or, more commonly calcaneo-varus or calcaneo-valgus in which the calcaneum has moved from its correct alignment with the lower leg.

This can be tested by the chiropodist who will measure the range of motion of the sub talar joint. Using a formula, the degree of calcaneal valgus/varus can be calculated. If the foot is still mobile, the chiropodist may provide stabilising functional orthoses, using the result obtained to adjust the orthotic to limit the range of motion. These are made of rigid thermoplastic, moulded on a plaster cast of the foot. This is only possible if the forefoot can adapt to the new position of the calcaneum. If not, stabilising one joint will only produce pain elsewhere. If this is the case, soft insoles with padding to increase weight-bearing of the underloaded parts of the foot, can be fitted.

The major effect of rearfoot deformity is the secondary damage and deformity caused to the forefoot, which by its very structure is more susceptible to damage. The forefoot tends to follow the direction of movement of the rearfoot, especially when non-weightbearing. Under load, the forefoot cannot always do this and may excessively pronate or supinate in order to achieve full loading, thereby compensating for the rearfoot deformity.

The first ray (first cuneiform and metatarsal) is capable of more movement than the others and is plantarflexed in normal propulsion. It can become abnormally plantar- or dorsi-flexed in an attempt to compensate for abnormality elsewhere.

Forefoot deformities, or symptoms connected with them are by far the commonest presenting feature. Hallux valgus is the most easily recognised and is frequently the cause of considerable pain and inability to wear readily-available shoes without cutting or distorting them. The aetiology of hallux valgus is complex, and can involve hereditary factors, rearfoot deformity, whole foot deformities and footwear. The end result of hallux valgus usually includes deformities of the lesser toes, extra depth to the toe area as a result of these, as well as the extreme width of the forefoot. Force distribution is altered due to an inefficient first metatarso-phalangeal joint. The area under the second metatarso-phalangeal joint becomes overloaded, both in terms of the duration and magnitude of loading. This results in callousities, corns and possibly ulcers.

Toe deformities frequently become fixed, and even where some joint movement is possible, soft tissue changes and muscular action maintain the deformity. In retracted toes, the tips no longer touch the ground and the metatarso-phalangeal joints may be subluxed. Poorly fitting footwear can add to the problem by restricting the room available for toe movement.

As correction of toe deformities without surgical intervention is virtually impossible in the elderly, chiropodial treatment will have three objectives:

(i) To increase function if possible.
(ii) To protect areas of high pressure on both dorsal and plantar surfaces.
(iii) To increase weight-bearing of underloaded areas on the plantar surface.

All these approaches depend on adequate footwear.

Supplying small 'toe props' which fit under one or more lesser toes can help to hold toes out straight to relieve pressure and increase function. These can be made of leather-covered foam, or moulded *in situ* from silicone rubber. Both are removed at night or for bathing. The patient must therefore be able to apply and remove them, and this should be tested in the surgery.

Hammer toes, where the proximal interphalangeal joint is in fixed flexion, are a particularly common and painful problem. Lesions such as corns and ulcers appear on both the dorsal surface of this prominence and on toe tip. Usually there is also a corresponding corn or callous under the second metatarso-phalangeal joint. The treatment for the dorsum can be by means of a horseshoe-shaped pad, preferably removable, which is thicker than the height of the prominence, so that the shoe upper rests on the pad.

Another approach, which can include cushioning for both dorsum and apex is to make a latex rubber cover for the toe or toes, using a plaster model of the relevant toe(s). Using liquid latex and suitable padding a removable device is made.

This method is also frequently used for protecting painful bunions. In this case, the model is usually first covered with very thin leather, as this is more pleasant to wear.

If padding is required for both dorsal and plantar lesions, and the toes are relatively immobile, it is possible to make a 'glove' for the whole of the forefoot, incorporating both. The appliance is again made on a plaster cast. It has soft leather on inside and out, with the padding as a sandwich, and fits under hosiery inside the shoe.

Plantar lesions can be improved by the use of either removable padding, rigid or soft orthoses. Removeable padding, held in place by loops around the toes and dorsum, may be of limited use as people may not be able to manage to get the loops on and off their toes.

Soft insoles, made on a semi-rigid base, can incorporate differing densities of padding, to give support under some areas and cushioning for others as appropriate. They can be covered in a variety of materials, usually soft leather or a man-made equivalent where perspiration or incontinence is a problem. Chiropodists make insoles to individual prescription, to fit a particular shoe as well as the foot to ensure a correct relationship.

Sub-cutaneous soft tissue disorders These include sprains and strains, tenosynovitis, bursitis and plantar fasciitis. The chiropodial approach to all aseptic inflammatory conditions will be to identify the cause, treat it and the presenting problem, to prevent recurrence. For example, biomechanical defects may indicate the use of orthoses. Reduction of swelling by judicial use of strapping or other methods to give rest, and re-mobilisation following the acute phase will form part of treatment. Heat and cold therapy, ultrasound and lasers are all used by chiropodists to treat such problems.

Bursae, anatomical and adventitious, are found in the feet. In the elderly, bursae over the medial side of the first metatarso-phalangeal joint, especially where there is hallux valgus, are probably the most troublesome. In their aquiescent state they can be protected by the use of made-to-measure 'bunion shields' as described above. Bursae frequently become infected due to necrosis of the overlying skin, or injudicial treatment of corns. Any established sinus may have to be chemically cauterised to allow removal of the fibrous lining which will otherwise prevent healing.

Infected subcutaneous lesions can be managed by the chiropodist, usually in conjunction with a physician if there is need of antibiotic cover. The management follows the usual lines for infected lesions, followed by treatment of the underlying cause, or protection of the area to prevent recurrence.

Skin and nail disorders These are probably the lesions which most people (wrongly) consider to be the principal concern of the chiropodist. They are certainly the reason for which many people first attend a chiropodist.

Callous is a normal physiological response of skin, when subjected to excess stress. It can only be regarded as pathological when it causes pain, or masks underlying necrosis as in diabetic or rheumatoid arthritic feet. The chiropodial management of callous requires identification of the cause, which is usually friction or shearing stress. Ill-fitting footwear which allows the foot to slide and biomechanical defects are the usual cause of such stresses. Immediate treatment will include the debridement of the excess thickness using a scalpel. Local medicaments (e.g. salicylic acid collodion B.P.C.) may be applied if appropriate, as may a thin adhesive dressing.

Corns are another example of pathological hyperkeratosis. Here, the area is very localised, frequently cone-shaped, with the point of the cone deepest in the skin. They are painful because the corn causes displacement of pain-sensitive nerve endings in the dermis. The cause is usually direct but intermittent pressure on a small area over a bony prominence. Once again, identification of the cause is the first step in treatment. This is followed by the removal of all the hard keratosis, followed by use of local medicaments, if appropriate, and the use of protective adhesive or removable padding. Corns are frequently considered intractable by patients, as they commonly recur. This is due to the cause either not being diagnosed, or being incurable. Poor footwear is frequently also to blame, as the chiropodist is prevented from providing adequate padding, temporary or permanent.

Dermatitis, psoriasis and many other skin disorders may manifest in the feet and the chiropodist is trained to treat the local problems, and may in fact be the first to detect systemic disorders through their effects on the feet.

Blisters, usually relatively trivial, can be the portal of entry for infection which can be severe in debilitated skin, through age, diabetes or other systemic diseases, and need careful attention.

Infections of the skin and nails are also treated by chiropodists. The only common viral infection of the foot is the wart or verruca. These are relatively rare in the elderly, usually pain-free, and may not be treated, unless they are getting larger, more numerous, or where there is danger of infecting others. Treatments include cryotherapy and electrosurgery as well as chemical treatments. Fungal infections are more common. Everyone carries dermatophytes on their skin, and several species cause flagrant athletes' foot, with characteristic itching, peeling between the toes, and spreading patches on more exposed surfaces. Treatment is with local medicaments, which must be continued for three to four weeks after symptoms have resolved, to prevent reinfection. In severe or recurrent cases, the footwear will have to be fumigated.

Bacterial infections are by far the commonest, ranging from superficial, short-term sepsis caused by minor trauma to acute infections of ulcers, leading to cellulitis or gangrene. The interdigital spaces carry not only dermatophyte fungi, but also staphylococcus aureus and β haemolytic streptococcus bacteria. Both cause potentially life-threatening infections, particularly in the debilitated or elderly patient. Bacterial infections include paronychia (infection around the nail) and onychia (infection of the nail matrix). Both may be caused by bacterial or fungal infection. Treatment will include identification of the causative organism, and follow the standard routine for infected lesions.

Ulcers, far from rare in the feet may be uninfected or infected, traumatic, neuropathic or vascular in origin. The uninfected type, caused by pressure, frequently under untreated callousities in debilitated feet, are prone to infection once the overlying callousity has been removed. Diabetics and rheumatoid patients are particularly liable to develop such lesions, and they may blame the chiropodist for causing the ulcer, as they are usually unaware of its presence prior to chiropody treatment. The aetiology of these ulcers is complex, including factors of circulatory and neuropathic origin. Any ulcer which has calloused or fibrous edges will be slow to heal, and the chiropodist can help by removing this tissue. Ulcer management by debridement, cleansing, local antiseptics and protective padding are everyday practice. Co-operation with the physician will be needed for antibiotic cover if appropriate, possible bed rest or diagnostic tests such as X-rays to eliminate or confirm possible diagnoses such as osteomyelitis.

Toenail disorders can be grouped into three groups: damage by trauma, by infection, or as a consequence of systemic disease. Damage by trauma is probably the commonest in elderly people. Very thick nails which grow long (onychogryphosis) are usually due to a major trauma to the nail matrix. Nails which grow thick but not particularly long or distorted (onychauxis) are thought to be caused by repeated minor traumata over a period of time, such as the wearing of too short shoes, which cause the toes to impact on the toe box. The conservative treatment is regular reduction with a nail drill to maintain a near normal thickness. This is a painless procedure, and necessary to prevent the development of sub-ungual ulceration.

Ingrown nails, where the skin has been breached by the nail (onychocryptosis) are most common in young men, but may be found in older people, usually due to incorrect nail cutting, which has left a rough edge onto which the flesh has been pushed by shoe pressure or other trauma. Conservative treatment includes removal of the offending portion of nail, treatment of any accompanying infection, and education to prevent recurrence. More radical treatment, for all three conditions, performed under local anaesthesia, involves surgical or chemical destruction of part or all of the nail matrix to prevent regrowth. This is a permanent cure, but may not be accepted by the patient, even if they are medically suitable for the procedure. Assessment of suitability may include testing of ankle/brachial index, along with routine urine testing and clinical examination.

Excessive curvature of the nails (viewed from toe tip) is probably hereditary or, possibly, caused by long-term lateral pressure from footwear. Pain is caused when footwear presses onto the dorsum of the nail, pushing the edges onto the flesh. There are a variety of treatments available, although attention to footwear is the most efficacious.

Nail problems may also indicate the presence of a sub-ungual exostosis, visible on X-ray and requiring minor surgery for removal.

Infection of toenails is by dermatophyte fungi. It can spread from or to the surrounding skin, or affect just the nail plate. Griseofulvin, the systemic treatment for fungal infections takes a period of about nine months as it only affects new nail growth. Patients may fail to take medication daily for such a long period and thus experience failure. Commonly, treatment is topical, for a period of at least nine months, with or without prior removal of the nail plate.

Psoriasis is one example of a systemic disease which causes nail damage, as they become thickened, pitted and crumbly.

Manifestations of systemic disorders

Whilst all systemic disorders have an effect on the structures of the feet, there are specific groups of disorders which put the feet at a higher risk of severe complications. These are:

— diabetes mellitus
— vascular disease
— disorders of the nervous system
— diseases requiring steroid therapy
— inflammatory joint disease

Diabetes causes macro and microangioathy, peripheral neuropathy and also carries a higher risk of atherosclerosis. The reduction of the blood supply to the skin reduces its viability and, when trauma or infections occur, the inflammatory response is impaired. Where there is diminished blood flow this causes lower oxygen perfusion, and toxin removal is slower. Systemic antibiotics and other drugs are less able to reach the site of infection. Healing times are lengthened, and in severe cases tissue necrosis occurs which may result in ulcers, or pre-gangrenous areas. Gangrene may develop, resulting in the loss of part or all of the foot or limb. Large vessel disease may further complicate the picture as this reduces the total blood flow to the limb.

The presence of peripheral neuropathy (with or without accompanying reduction in blood flow) in the diabetic increases the risk from trauma, as blisters and minor abrasions may go unnoticed, unless hosiery or footwear is bloodstained. As many diabetics have retinopathy, this too can be unobserved. The necessary daily inspection of the feet and footwear should be carried out by a carer if the diabetic cannot do so. Examination of the patient by any member of the team should include all surfaces of the feet with hosiery removed. Sensory neuropathy increases the risk of pressure-related ulceration, as the person will not shift weight from overloaded areas, as do those with normal sensation even when standing still. When the motor nerves become involved, there is an alteration in the digital function, leading to abnormal foot function. Autonomic neuropathy affects circulation and can lead to arterio-venous shunting and a reduction in the activity of the sweat glands.

Peripheral vascular disease can also occur in the non-diabetic, from a variety of causes. The effect on the skin is similar, with the feet needing protection from rough seams in hosiery and footwear.

In the same way, peripheral neuropathy may be present with other disorders, including pernicious anaemia, alcohol abuse, polio (motor only) and spina bifida, for example. Loss of motor nerves results in loss of reflexes and muscle wasting. There is a reduction in the blood supply, with consequent effects on healing times and skin health. Gait is affected, with foot drop being common. When combined with loss of proprioception, damage to skin and subcutaneous structures including the joints occurs.

Steroids suppress the inflammatory response to local trauma by the skin and soft tissues, increasing the risk from infections. Osteoporosis, always a potential problem in the very elderly and particularly women, can be exacerbated or caused by the use of steroid drugs.

The principles of treatment of all high-risk feet are similar to those for all feet, but with greater emphasis on diagnosis, examination and patient education. More investigations than usual may be undertaken such as doppler ultrasound for circulation, X-rays and swabs for the earliest identification of pathogens. Treatments are more conservative as poor healing power may contraindicate radical measures but the treatment of infections is even more intensive. There is great emphasis on prevention of complications. Education of the patient and/or their carers is particularly important, as early detection of a problem can make a great difference in the prognosis. High-risk feet call for an even greater degree of teamwork, with the professionals, patient and carers working together.

FOOTWEAR

Footwear, which in this context includes slippers, sandals, shoes and boots, plays a vital role in the care of the feet, and the maintenance of mobility. There are basic requirements for well-fitting footwear which apply to all adults, not just the elderly. These are generally poorly understood by all sections of the community, and are given here as a basic guide to a very complex subject.

Fitting points

Length Closed-fronted shoes should allow 1.25 cm gap between the end of the longest toe and the shoe front.

Width Must be adequate across both the ball of the foot and the toes.

Depth The uppers should not press down on the toes.

Fastening If the foot is not to slip forward into the necessary gap at the front of the shoe, there must be an adjustable fastening across the instep. Laces, bars with buckles, 'velcro' (touch and close fabric), are all adequate. Specialist fastenings such as hooks or ski boot fastenings can be useful in particular cases. Zips are not ideal, as they do not allow for feet that swell, but are better than no fastening, especially on slippers.

Heels Should be thick, and no higher than 3.75 cm. If there is ankle equinus or pain in the calves when standing barefoot, flat shoes are to be avoided.

Material There is little doubt that leather is the material of preference, but some of today's plastics are nearly as pliable, and can be better if incontinence is a problem.

For many elderly people, especially women, the shoes easily available in the High Street shops are unsuitable, often because of lack of forefoot width and of fastenings. It is true that women (in the United Kingdom at least) have far more foot problems than their male contemporaries, and there are more elderly women than men. The problem is compounded by the fact that most women's shoes are not foot-shaped, whilst the majority of shoes for men are much closer to the natural shape, and frequently have laces. There are some shoe companies which specialise in wide-fitting shoes, aimed at the older consumer, who trade through retail shops, but these are usually only suitable for the less-deformed feet. If the woman has fairly large feet, it may be possible to obtain lace-up shoes in the mens' department, now that there is a blurring of design differences. This can be true of slippers, or if a trainer style is acceptable. Some independent retailers (the small family-type of business) are particularly helpful in this area, and it is worth locating your nearest shop to investigate what they can offer.

Chain-store shoes should not be dismissed out of hand, as they do sometimes sell acceptable styles (in health terms), and are often within the price range of pensioners. They also have the advantage of being 'normal', which is very important psychologically. Likewise, trainers are not all bad, and can make excellent substitutes for slippers or outdoor shoes. Perspiration is rarely a problem, and some trainers are machine-washable. They frequently have flared heels which add lateral stability.

If it is not possible to purchase shoes in the High Street shops, then consideration must be given to the other sources and types of footwear. There are now semi-orthopaedic shoes available for purchase or prescribable on the NHS. These shoes are built on special lasts which give extra depth and width to the shoes. Loose insoles are frequently included which can be removed and replaced with purpose-made ones. The shoes are only partly made to measure, the fitting taking place using a 'standard' shoe. Any alterations which are needed are noted and the actual shoes ordered from the manufacturer in the colour required. There is a time delay but this is not usually as long as for wholly made-to-measure shoes. The cost is lower as some of the components are mass-produced.

Bespoke shoes, made-to-measure for each foot, can be purchased privately or obtained through the NHS on prescription. They are very expensive as shoe-making is very labour intensive, many of the operations being done by hand. They are the only answer for very deformed feet, or where there is great difference in foot size. There can be considerable delays in the supply of these shoes and patients may be discharged from hospital long before the shoes arrive. They can also be rather heavy for frail people as DHSS contracts specify the standard to which the shoes must conform. It is important at the measuring stage to check that the patient will be able to put on and remove the shoes, with or without the use of a dressing stick, or have someone who will be able to do so daily. It is not unusual to find that this is not the case.

In order to speed rehabilitation, it is important that the patient is wearing either their usual shoes, a good temporary shoe, or their prescribed footwear. The patient's carer (or social worker, etc.) can be asked to bring in a selection of owned footwear in order to use the most suitable pair. An industrial shoe-stretcher can facilitate speedy minor alterations especially when post-operative oedema makes only one foot swollen. If nothing suitable exists, many relatives will be willing to purchase a new pair if given guidance as to what to buy. Some rehabilitation units or long-stay institutions may have their own store, shop or links with suitable suppliers.

Temporary shoes come in a variety of styles, from the orthopaedic sandal, through to the plastazote shoe which has a proper sole and uppers which are heat mouldable with a hair drier. Felt shoes, machine-washable are available, but are unsuitable for incontinent patients as the felt readily soaks up urine.

To aid walking, shoes must be well-fitting, allow the insertion of any orthoses prescribed, be comfortable and look attractive. The first point is to ensure that the shoes do not inhibit gait by slipping or adding to the patients' feeling of instability. It is important that the chiropodist be included in the consultation prior to the purchase or measuring for shoes. The combination of doctor, orthotist, chiropodist and psysiotherapist should produce the best result.

Comfort is extremely important to the patient, and may be a major factor in gaining acceptance of the shoes. If patients are used to light and sloppy slippers, they may find shoes too stiff and heavy initially. Their skin, unused to contact with a shoe, may feel sore even if there are no visible signs. Short periods of wear, even whilst sitting still, can help to accustom the patient to them. Soles which do not slip and thereby allow shuffling will also cause some problems unless a re-educative programme of gait training is simultaneously undertaken.

Appearance is probably the factor most frequently overlooked and undervalued by prescribers, and the most important to the patient. No-one, however old, wants to wear something which marks them out as different or abnormal. Colour can play an important part and the lighter colours now available are often more acceptable. The restriction to two or three pairs of prescribed shoes poses problems particularly for women, who generally have a far larger number and variety of shoes than their male contemporaries.

STATE REGISTERED CHIROPODISTS AND HOW TO REFER

All chiropodists employed by the NHS have to be on the current State Register, published annually. The designatory letters are SRCh. They may also be members of the Society of Chiropodists (MChS). At present, the Society is the only organisation whose training and examinations are approved for the purposes of State Registration. There are other organisations who train chiropodists who are only able to practice in the voluntary and private sectors. The training to become State Registered is a three-year, full-time course, and the topics studied include physiology, anatomy, biomechanics and gait, pharmacology, medicine, surgery, and the practical treatment of most foot conditions. The use of injectable local anaesthetics is also included. These prescription-only drugs are only available to registered chiropodists who hold the appropriate certificate.

The State Registered Chiropodist is trained to diagnose and treat almost all foot conditions. They are also trained to recognise many other conditions, both specific to the foot and of many general or systemic disorders which require referral to a specialist medical practitioner.

There are only about 6,000 State Registered Chiropodists in the United Kingdom, and the whole-time equivalent of about half that number work for the NHS. The spread of chiropodists is not even geographically, with the result that some health districts are much better served than others. This, along with differing organisational policies explains why there may be long waiting lists for treatment. In addition, whilst much can be done to relieve the older person from foot pain, they usually require some form of continuing care with the result that the chiropodist soon reaches the point of maximum case load and cannot take any further patients without lengthening the interval between treatments. The basic norm for NHS chiropodists is 500 patients, of which about 400 will be elderly, if treatment is to be given at an *average* of six weeks. In terms of population, it is generally assumed that there should be one chiropodist per 1,000 elderly persons in the community. With an elderly population of almost 12,000,000, the United Kingdom has only half the State Registered Chiropodists needed.

Some Health Authorities also employ Foot Care Assistants (or Chiropody Assistants) who carry out simple tasks such as nail cutting, and assisting the chiropodist in the surgery. These people provide a useful service to many disabled or elderly people whose problem is simply that they cannot manage their own nails. Screening by a chiropodist will occur before referral to a foot care assistant, and usually at suitable intervals thereafter. A chiropodist with access to a foot care assistant will therefore be able to carry a larger than normal case load.

Anyone can refer a person to a chiropodist. Within the NHS there may be local rules such as in some hospitals which restrict referral to consultants or their teams. Some Health Authorities provide treatments only in clinics or hospitals, whilst others have mobile surgeries or provide transport to bring the less mobile to a clinic. Some provide domiciliary visits, but these pose some problems of instrument sterilisation and are very time-consuming which again reduces the chiropodists' case load.

It is possible to have private treatment from State Registered Chiropodists as well as from the non-registered. Fees vary and domiciliary visits may be expensive because of the travel costs involved. (It is wise to check before committing oneself.) The various chiropodial organisations will give names of local private chiropodists to enquirers and it is always possible to check the State Register at the local reference library. Many Yellow Pages Telephone Directories now contain a separate entry for State Registered Chiropodists.

REFERENCES

Cartwright, A. and Henderson, G. (1987) *More Trouble with Feet*. HMSO, London

Clarke, M. (1969) *Trouble with Feet*. Bell, London

Kemp, J. and Winkler, J.T. (1983) *Problems Afoot: Need and Efficiency Footcare*. Disabled Living Foundation, London

9

Rehabilitation and Elderly Ethnic Minorities

James George and John Young

INTRODUCTION

The elders of ethnic minorities face a potential triple jeopardy: at risk through old age, through discrimination and through lack of access to health and social services (Norman 1985). Traditionally, Britain has accepted a variety of ethnic minority groups within its population so that many different races and cultures are represented in the United Kingdom elderly (Table 9.1). In some inner city areas the so-called ethnic minorities are in fact the majority and the number of their elderly is increasing. In order to provide good care we need to be aware of the background and special health problems and requirements of the ethnic minority groups.

DEFINITION

The term ethnic minority group is used to refer to people of any race who see themselves as sharing a common culture which is distinct from that of the majority of the population as a whole.

BACKGROUND OF SOME ETHNIC MINORITY GROUPS

Elderly people of Polish origin

At the turn of this century many Polish Jews came to the United Kingdom fleeing persecution. They settled mainly in the East End of London, Manchester and Leeds and tend to speak Polish or Yiddish.

Table 9.1: People of pensionable age resident in the United Kingdom by country of birth (thousands)

United Kingdom	9,063.2
Irish Republic	132.0
Old Commonwealth (includes Australia, Canada and New Zealand)	21.3
New Commonwealth:	
East Africa (includes Kenya, Malawi, Tanzania, Uganda and Zambia)	1.6
Rest of Africa	1.1
Caribbean (includes Barbados, Jamaica, Trinidad, Tobago, Belize and Guyana)	16.2
Bangladesh	3.8
India	44.1
Far East	3.9
Mediterranean (includes Cyprus, Gibraltar, Malta and Gozo)	3.7
Pakistan	4.8
European Community	41.8
Other foreigners	113.5

Source: Census 1981

After the Second World War 100,000 members of the Polish forces stayed in Britain and there were also many wartime refugees. Most of these Poles settled in London, Birmingham, Manchester and Bradford, with smaller populations in Wolverhampton, Leeds, Nottingham, Sheffield, Coventry, Leicester and Slough. The post-war Polish settlers are mostly Roman Catholic, although some are Jews.

Elderly people of Indian origin

People came to the United Kingdom from two main Indian states: Punjab and Gujarat. The men came in the 1950s and early 1960s and were joined by their families, often many years later.

People from the Indian Punjab speak Punjabi and most are Sikh by religion. There are large Punjabi Sikh communities in the West Midlands, Glasgow, West London and Leeds.

People of Gujarati origin from India and East Africa live mainly in North and South London, Coventry, Leicester and Manchester. Most are Hindus.

The national language of India is Hindi but relatively few people

157

of Indian origin speak Hindi as a first language; many speak it as a second language.

Elderly people of Pakistani origin

Many people from Pakistan came to Britain during the late 1950s and early 1960s. They came from three main areas — Mirpur in Azad (Free) Kashmir, Punjab province and North West Frontier Province. As well as their regional language, they will probably speak Urdu. Most people of Pakistani origin live in Yorkshire, Lancashire, Greater Manchester, West Midlands, Cardiff and Glasgow. The majority of Pakistanis are Muslim.

Elderly people of Bangledeshi origin

Most people from Bangladesh came to the United Kingdom in the 1950s and 1960s and settled throughout the country, but especially in the East End of London. Most Indian restaurants are staffed by Bangladeshis. Almost all are Muslim and come from the rural Sylhet district of Bangladesh and speak a Sylheti dialect.

Elderly people of Vietnamese origin

Vietnamese refugees are recent migrants. Several thousand Vietnamese now live in Britain and may have come via refugee camps in Hong Kong. The majority came from North Vietnam and most are ethnic Chinese who speak both Cantonese and Vietnamese. They may become isolated as many are in rural areas, far from other Vietnamese families.

Elderly people of Afro-Caribbean origin

The great majority of elderly people from the West Indies came to the United Kingdom in the boom period after the Second World War. Many intended originally to return home. Over half the West Indians who came to Britain came from Jamaica: others came from Guyana, Barbados, Trinidad and Tobago. As with other groups, they tend to be concentrated in inner city areas. However, compared to the other groups, they tend to be very stable in terms of domicile with a high rate of council house occupation rather than being owner-occupiers (Barker 1984). It is important to remember that there are very distinct differences in culture and previous experience between people from different islands in the Caribbean. Many West Indians are Christians; the largest group are Pentecostalists, some are Anglicans or Baptists and a few are Methodists or Roman Catholics.

HOUSING AND SOCIAL ASPECTS OF ETHNIC MINORITIES

Most of the ethnic minority elders are concentrated in the inner and middle centres of cities where environmental problems are most acute. Asian and Afro-Caribbean households are more likely to live in older housing and to suffer overcrowding (Barker 1984).

Ethnic minority elders tend to be concentrated in unskilled and semi-skilled occupations where they are more vulnerable to unemployment. Consequently they tend to rely on minimum state pensions and may live close to the poverty line. Furthermore, language difficulties may make it difficult for ethnic minority elders to receive the appropriate social and housing benefits. It is tempting to assume that support by the close-knit family network of ethnic minorities can in some way compensate for these disadvantages. Unfortunately, this does not seem to be so and the pattern of elderly parents living with their children appears to be changing (Blakemore 1983). There seems to be a need for more sheltered housing (Age Concern 1984) and more day centres for ethnic minority groups (Norman 1985). (The booklet *Which Benefit?* (FB2) is available in Urdu, Gujarati, Hindi, Punjabi, Bengali and Chinese, as well as English and should be available in all departments treating elderly ethnic minority patients.)

MEDICAL ASPECTS

There has been comparatively little research on the particular medical problems of elderly ethnic minority patients. Asian patients are known to be more likely to suffer from ischaemic heart disease

159

and there may be more delay in their being transferred to Coronary Care Units from Casualty, presumably because of language difficulties (Lawrence and Littler 1985). In one London hospital casualty department it was found that 69 (12 per cent) of all patients seen in one week did not have a good command of English (Dawson *et al.* 1983). Only 19 (28 per cent) of these patients attended with an outside interpreter, usually a friend or relative. Often these outside 'interpreters' were little better than the patients in command of English.

Myocardial infarctions seem to be less common in Afro-Caribbeans but this group seem more likely to suffer hypertension and strokes (Beevers and Cruickshank 1981).

A survey in Birmingham of 342 Afro-Caribbean and Asian elderly revealed that both groups seemed more likely than the indigenous elderly to have visited their general practitioner during the preceding six months (Blakemore 1983).

Donaldson (1986) surveyed 726 Asian elderly over 65 in Leicester. He found that over half the Asian elderly over-75s were not independent in activities of daily living and one fifth had some urinary incontinence. These findings, however, do not differ greatly from those for the non-Asian population. One major difference was that more Asian over-75s were able to bathe independently than non-Asian elderly (82 per cent compared to 62 per cent). Perhaps this is because of different methods of bathing, as many Asians prefer to shower rather than sit in a bath. Donaldson also found that only 37 per cent of Asian elderly men and 2 per cent of Asian elderly women were able to speak English. A handful (4 per cent) of Asian elderly were living alone compared to 46 per cent of non-Asians. Only half of the Asians interviewed were familiar with Meals-on-Wheels or home helps, and very few were receiving any social service help. Nearly 90 per cent were not aware of the chiropody service and only 3 per cent were receiving chiropody help.

GENERAL APPROACH TO ETHNIC MINORITY PATIENTS IN HOSPITAL

Irrespective of cultural background, illness brings anxiety and distress for the individual and family. Nevertheless, for some ethnic minority patients admitted to hospital, unfamiliarity with the system and separation from their family home and culture can exaggerate the upset involved with illness. This can be potentiated by staff who have insufficient knowledge to modify their approach to suit the differing needs of these patients.

Hindu, Muslim and Sikh women are embarrassed at having to expose areas of their body. Legs and upper arms should remain covered at all times. Consequently, hospital 'nightgowns' may be especially humiliating. Modesty should be maintained as far as possible during nursing procedures and physiotherapy or occupational therapy treatment sessions. Careful explanation, if necessary through an interpreter, tact and negotiation of the most appropriate and acceptable method of performing a task should be the aim. This also fosters a spirit of understanding and concern which helps minimise feelings of isolation or distress engendered by the hospital admission. This is particularly valuable if the patient has a disabling condition as the framework will be laid for the necessary close co-operation (often for a long period) between staff and patient. Irritation, impatience and intolerance will be counter-productive and ultimately undermine the rehabilitation process. It should be borne in mind that the feelings of modesty are deeply ingrained and cannot be easily overcome by simple willpower. Sympathy and understanding are required.

Similar respect should be paid to religious needs, jewellery, diet and hygiene requirements. Asian patients may prefer to wash in free-flowing water rather than sit in a bath. Hospitals in many developing countries expect the family to undertake much of the basic care. Illness is shared and generally one family member will always be present at the bedside. The British practice of restricted hospital visiting may need to be relaxed. It is essential to use the correct name for patients, including the personal name (e.g. 'Mr Rajinder Singh', not just 'Mr Singh').

Attitudes to ill-health also differ. Illness is sometimes regarded as something to be suffered, and it is the expected behaviour to remain 'ill' and in bed until full recovery has occurred. Thus, illnesses in which full recovery may not occur (e.g. stroke, arthritis) may need particularly careful management. The concept of active rehabilitation may be unfamiliar to many elderly ethnic minority patients.

Sometimes there may be conflict in the family between the elders with traditional views and the children who have become 'Westernised' and may expect the State to provide much of the care. Occasionally, residential care may be regarded with suspicion and arrangements should be made for patients to visit a residential home before deciding whether this is an option.

COMMUNICATION ACROSS A LANGUAGE BARRIER

Rehabilitation is a highly active process where the onus of responsibility of recovery is transferred from the rehabilitation staff to the patient. It involves the patient re-learning old tasks or making adjustments to allow a new way of life. Two items are essential. Firstly, the patient and family should gain an understanding of the disabling condition and its consequences. This is essentially an education process. Secondly, the patient and family will need to be actively involved in a set of often complex manoeuvres to maximise recovery of the damaged body system. Adequate communication is the key to success for both these tasks. Many elderly ethnic minority patients, particularly Asians and East Europeans, will have lived in enclaves of their own cultures. Their knowledge of English will consequently be non-existent or rudimentary. Potentially, this produces a major barrier to successful rehabilitation and represents an important initial task for the staff planning rehabilitation programmes.

There are several practical ways in which rehabilitation staff can improve communication with people who speak little or no English. Ideally, it should be possible to use a qualified interpreter who has had training and is skilled in the nuances of the technique. Every hospital should have a list of locally available interpreters. A good interpreter is more than just a translator. He must form a relationship with the patient and provide a bridge between two cultures and two sets of expectations. If a qualified interpreter is not available, relatives and friends may be able to help. This has the additional advantage that the family become closely involved with the rehabilitation programme and are in a better position to maintain recovery following discharge from the hospital. However, a degree of care is needed as sometimes sensitive problems will be encountered which the patient will be reluctant or unwilling to communicate details through someone he knows. If no interpreter is available, it is important that staff take a little more time to check that instructions are understood, observing the points listed in Table 9.2.

Table 9.2: Ways to improve communication

Use a qualified interpreter if possible
Simplify your English
Speak slowly and be patient
Give non-verbal reassurance
Get the patient's name right and pronounce it correctly
Keep comprehensive records to avoid repetition
Check back — check instructions by asking the patient to explain back to
  you what he is going to do
Try and avoid questions in which the correct answer is simply 'Yes'
Avoid idioms (e.g. 'spend a penny')
Write down important points on a piece of paper for the patient to take
  away

TEAMWORK

The essence of rehabilitation of the elderly requires teamwork and plenty of time. Valued additional members of the team may be a social worker or health visitor with a specific expertise in caring for ethnic minority patients, and also an interpreter (*vide supra*). All members of the team may need to spend more time explaining the aims of therapy and the likely outcome to both the patient and family. A home visit may be invaluable to set aims and objectives and to ensure that improvement is maintained after discharge. A checklist of points for all members of the rehabilitation team to consider is given in Table 9.3.

COMMON CONDITIONS

Stroke

Stroke illness makes demands at all levels of health and social service and also tests family relationships, whatever the culture. There are many common misapprehensions about stroke (Table 9.4) which may hamper recovery and need to be tackled. More leaflets and videos about stroke illness in different languages are required. The setting up of more stroke clubs to cater for ethnic minorities may also help.

Table 9.3: Checklist for rehabilitation staff

Communication
Has the following been explained? (Use an interpreter if necessary)
  — Instructions about medication
  — Implications of illness and likely recovery
  — Need for further tests
  — Roles of various therapists
  — Aims of rehabilitation therapy
  — Follow up arrangements

Religion
Are there particular religious requirements?
  — Formal prayer
  — Fasting

Diet
Are there particular dietary requirements?
  — Vegetarian
  — Halal meat

Hygiene
Are there particular hygiene requirements?
  — Running water for washing
  — Ritual washing
  — Use of left hand for toilet and right for eating

Social
Is the patient receiving the appropriate social benefits?
  — State or private pension
  — Attendance allowance
  — Mobility allowance

Table 9.4: False beliefs about stroke

Strokes are the same as heart attacks
Strokes are a punishment
The patient can get better just as quickly as they became ill
Exercise is bad for the hemiplegic side
The patient needs plenty of rest until complete recovery occurs
Physiotherapists, occupational therapists and speech therapists are types of nurse
Treatment of strokes is mainly tablets from the doctor
Relatives and friends can't help with treatment

Depression and dementia

Depression may be undertreated in ethnic minority patients as it is often difficult to diagnose and may present with more physical symptoms. Depression may prevent a patient reaching his or her full potential and may be more readily detected by nurses and therapists who spend longer periods in close contact with the individual patients, than do doctors. Likewise, dementia is less easily diagnosed, as the family may be less forthcoming with the symptoms of personality change and memory impairment. Psychological tests can be misleading as they are dependent on language ability and educational background.

Amputations

Leg amputations may be very much less easy to accept in some ethnic minority groups. This is because it implies disfigurement and loss of income. Patients may not be aware of the possibilities of achieving independence and a good quality of life following the operation — with appropriate help. Effective counselling and a positive approach may help to overcome these problems.

RECOMMENDATIONS TO IMPROVE CARE OF ELDERLY ETHNIC MINORITY PATIENTS

The many ethnic minority groups have widely differing needs and it is therefore difficult to make general recommendations. However, the following five points should be considered:

(i) Teaching about ethnic minority elderly patients to be included in the training of all health professionals.

(ii) More health education leaflets, books and videos to be available in different languages to help explain the facilities already available.

(iii) More specialist workers for ethnic minority patients, e.g. specialist health visitors, social workers, community physiotherapists and occupational therapists.

(iv) More stroke clubs and day centres for ethnic minority groups.

(v) More research into the needs of ethnic minority elderly patients at both a local and national level.

SUMMARY

Elderly ethnic minority patients come from widely diverse backgrounds and have a wide variety of different needs. Every patient should be treated as an individual but understanding of the various backgrounds, religions and cultures will help to improve medical management and rehabilitation.

Fundamentally the same sympathetic concern, attention to detail, perseverance and patience are needed, as that required to care for other elderly patients. Further research is required into the needs of this important and increasing group of elderly people.

REFERENCES

Age Concern/Help the Aged Housing Trust (1984). *Housing for Ethnic Elders*. Age Concern, Mitcham

Barker, J. (1984) *Black and Asian Old People in Britain*. Age Concern, Mitcham

Beevers, D.G. and Cruickshank, J.K. (1981) Age, sex, ethnic origin and hospital admission for heart attack and stroke. *Postgraduate Medical Journal, 57*, 763–5

Blakemore, K. (1983) Ethnicity, self-reported illness and use of medical services by the elderly. *Postgraduate Medical Journal, 59*, 668–70

Dawson, A.G., Hildrey, A.C.C. and Floyer, M.A. (1983) Health problems of ethnic minorities. *British Medical Journal, 286*, 1575–6

Donaldson, L.J. (1986) Health and social status of elderly Asians: a community survey. *British Medical Journal, 293*, 1079–82

Lawrence, R.E. and Littler, W.A. (1985) Acute myocardial infarction in Asians and Whites in Birmingham. *British Medical Journal, 290*, 1472

Norman, A. (1985) *Triple Jeopardy: Growing Old in a Second Homeland*. Centre for Policy on Ageing, London

10

Social Work with Elderly People

Alison Froggatt

To contribute a chapter to this book, highlighting the part social work plays in helping to rehabilitate elderly people, is valuable, as this kind of practice does not receive priority within social service departments. This is because of the heavy demands for social work with children and families, despite there being a large number of old people in the United Kingdom. 'By 1988 those over 75 will comprise one in 15 of the total population' (Phillipson and Walker 1986). Any elderly person who can be successfully rehabilitated to continue independent life for a period, is not only improving his/her quality of life, but continuing to make a contribution to society as a whole.

This chapter focuses on communication and co-operation. Communication is a key activity in social work. The skills lie in understanding and collecting information, facts or feelings, about the patient and family, and disseminating that information appropriately, and confidently, to members of the multidisciplinary team, the patient, relatives and/or other carers. Co-operation is emphasised because many different skills are required; rehabilitation is a shared activity, as this book demonstrates, including members of the primary health care and social service teams in the community. (I am writing about social work for the non-social work team members, and for social workers who may be new to practice in a rehabilitation setting, beginning with hospital-based work, then refer-ring to community-based work in area offices.)

Social workers are not asked to see every patient, but to participate with social or emotional problems, combining individualising the patient and his/her problem, to help him/her find a way through it, with obtaining and setting up resources to assist in resolving that problem. There are broadly counselling and social care planning functions. Other kinds of social work involve family work with patients and relatives, group work activities for elderly people and/or their relatives, and resource creation, networking in the community to provide more local resources (Sinclair 1984).

SOCIAL WORK PRACTICE IN A REHABILITATION SETTING

Social work with patients presupposes that there has been some illness or injury, resulting in an impairment, bodily or mental, with functional disability, and possibly a handicap in terms of role (Bury 1979). These technical terms are an aid to thinking clearly. The impairment could be a stroke, broken leg, chest infection, or memory loss; how far will it leave a permanent loss of function, even after rehabilitation of various sorts? Will the old lady with a right-sided stroke be able to learn to cook with her left hand? How far will she be handicapped in the role she expects to play in the home? Functional assessment, and remedial treatment are provided by the rehabilitation team as a group.

Whether the elderly patient is in hospital or has returned home, any member of the rehabilitation team can refer the person to the social service department, through the hospital-based social workers, or directly to the area team where the patient lives. Usually close relationships build up between multidisciplinary colleagues, despite differences in priorities, and approaches. Sometimes a social service team in a hospital operates an intake system, taking referrals in turn from every part of the hospital. This way of working offers a more consistent emergency service but makes it harder for social workers to build up expertise, in particular areas of work.

Where it is hoped to rehabilitate an elderly person to return home, early referral to the social worker is helpful, giving time to the patient and principal relatives, to establish the pattern of life before illness, and work out alterations needed to help the patient live at home. Sometimes one finds that the situation at home had been very difficult, or the stronger spouse is the one who has collapsed. Families might rule out the possibility of a return home and take action, such as giving up a flat, or making alternative and permanent arrangements for the remaining spouse; early discussion helps to keep the situation fluid. This kind of discussion is frequently initiated by members of the rehabilitation team, as part of their care plan; co-operation is needed to avoid duplication, and burdening relatives with excessive anxiety. As social workers become thinner on the ground in rehabilitation work, because of other demands, this aspect of their work may get overlooked. Yet to play a full part in assessment, counselling and social care planning, an early under-standing of the situation is helpful.

The next section explores welfare provisions, and other background knowledge helpful to think through before meeting the patient. Facilities and services for old people are available from all the main sectors of welfare provision, statutory, voluntary, informal care (meaning family and friends) and from the commercial or private sector.

STATUTORY SERVICES

Statutory provisions for old people are laid down in Acts of Parlia-ment, and given substance through the work of social service depart-ments and health authorities. The legal framework for old people has been discussed fully elsewhere in a valuable work, *The Law and Vulnerable Elderly People* (Age Concern 1986), and I have given (in Appendix I) details of the various legislation currently in place. Here we look briefly at some of the more pertinent Acts. The Social Services Act, 1970, established social service departments for each local authority, incorporating the Children's Department and the Welfare Departments responsible for mental welfare and old peoples' welfare. Medical social workers had been distributed unevenly through the hospitals. It was hoped when social service departments took over social workers for hospitals in 1972, that a more equitable service would result. Now in area offices within the larger hospitals, with an accountability to the social service department, social workers may be required to continue statutory work for infants and children discharged home, in the interests of continuity of worker for those families. This cuts into the time available for meeting the needs of current hospital patients.

Local authority social workers are employed in local government departments; in a managerial sense they are accountable to the senior social worker, or team leader, to the area officer, up to the Director of Social Services, who is in turn appointed by, and accountable to, the councillors on the social services committee. Social service departments tend to be divided into functions — field work, domiciliary care, and residential care with subdivisions for client groups, namely child care, mentally ill and handicapped people, old and disabled people. In negotiating for a particular client, e.g. a place in a residential home, social workers are competing for resources through a set of procedures which try to ensure fairness.

Residential care is the most expensive provision for elderly people. It takes 55 per cent of the total social service cost, the home help service 31 per cent, day care 4 per cent, Meals-on-Wheels 3 per cent, sheltered housing 4 per cent, other services 3 per cent (Audit Commission 1985) so deciding how much residential care to provide, and whom to admit to it, are the crucial questions in allocating resources, but intensive community care can cost more than residential care (Audit Commission 1986).

Domiciliary services

Home Care Those in charge are often called Home Care Organisers, co-ordinating a range of tending services, which play a significant part in helping old people to remain at home. These services, depending on the locality, can include home helps, home care aides going into the same home three or four times a day, Meals-on-Wheels and a night-sitter service. Because of this expansion the home care organiser may have an increasingly major role as care manager for many old people (Latto 1982). However, we are still talking about a very small minority of elderly people; the main service on offer, home helps, reach 3 per cent of the people over 65, and 15 per cent of those over 75 (Levin *et al.* 1985). The rest continue to care for themselves, or manage with help from family and friends.

Meals-on-Wheels This service is often funded by the local authority, with the meals being cooked in their residential homes but being distributed by volunteers. In 1984 for example, 44,988,000 were distributed (Audit Commission 1986). This may still only work out at two meals a week for some old people. With the advent of frozen food, some meals may be distributed in bulk at less frequent intervals. This does not get over the problem that those most in need may forget to heat up a meal, and need a home help to come in and warm it up for them.

Aids and adaptations The provision of aids and adaptations through the work of community-based occupational therapists will be covered in Chapters 11 and 13. There can be some overlap between community-based social workers and occupational therapists, and close collaboration is often helpful in particular cases. The occupational therapist is acknowledged by the Audit Commission (1986) as central to community care policy, yet their report identifies only one worker for every 1,000 people in the community needing such care.

Sheltered housing This term covers purpose-built, or adapted, housing for old or disabled people, each flat equipped with an alarm linked to a residential warden, so that help is normally on hand. A warden usually makes a personal call every morning. Of elderly people, 5 per cent live in council-built sheltered housing (Tinker 1981). Wardens are also provided by many local authorities on a peripatetic basis, making daily visits to 20 or 30 elderly people in their locality. Residents eventually become increasingly frail, incontinent or forgetful, imposing an excessive burden on wardens, and may need to move into residential accommodation. The chance of an old person in changed circumstances obtaining sheltered housing quickly will vary from one local authority to another.

Fostering for elderly people

Fostering has been extended to other client groups, including old people. In a study of such schemes Ware (1983) found that 22 per cent of local authorities had made arrangements to provide short-stay breaks for old people in private family homes, for payment.

Ethnic minority elders

Initiatives have been taken by some local authorities with an increasing population of elderly people from ethnic minority groups, realising that residential and day care, Meals-on-Wheels, and the kind of home helps recruited need to be appropriate to the requirements of people with different customs. It is recognised that problems of poverty, and poor inner city housing, or having a couple both out at work, affect the whole population (Norman 1985). Recent examples of appropriate provision for ethnic minority elders include

171

reserving a wing of an old peoples' home for East European elderly people, with a bilingual social worker based there, and establishing a day centre that will regularly offer Halal meals. The employment of an Urdu-speaking home help organiser who might be able to recruit the kind of older woman who would be acceptable as a home help in a South Asian household, or a small group home as part of sheltered housing with an Urdu-speaking warden, are future possibilities to be implemented.

Residential care

Temporary or permanent residential care is provided by local authorities for disabled and elderly people, known as 'Part III' accommodation (see Appendix I). With the increase in numbers of very old people over 85 (and the average age of residents over 80 in many areas), emphasis is increasingly on careful rehabilitation and assessment to ensure that no-one is offered a place in residential care unnecessarily. Many of those in residential care are not those most heavily dependent (Audit Commission 1985). People can become too dependent for residential care yet still be maintained at home, as residential care is intended for those who are able to walk or manage a wheelchair to get around, and can partly dress themselves, but who are not needing more medical attention than they could get if living at home in the community. While residents may stay in a home if incontinence develops, admission with this condition is more problematic. In fact only 1.5 per cent of people over 65 are in such local authority homes (Parker 1985). Severely disabled residents needing aids and adaptations can create difficulties in a home. There is now an 'Officer in Charge' not a Matron, indicative of expectations on residents.

Residential care is society's main provision for elderly people who are considered to be unable to cope at home any more. Purpose-built homes have reduced the original old 'workhouse' stigma, but the environment is frequently one which offers little choice, individualisation and stimulation (Willcocks 1986).

Short-stay, or rotational respite, care offers a service so that elderly people can stay in their own homes, provided the principal carers can get regular breaks. Thus the old person is admitted to a residential home in a planned way; a person who is heavily dependent can be admitted for two weeks in every eight, or even spend three weeks in and three weeks at home. A study of the increasing use of short-stay care (Allen 1983) explores many of the issues around the use of this kind of care. Not all old people are happy to be whisked into residential care for a 'holiday', and a lucid old person placed with a group of muddled long-stay residents might be particularly unhappy. Allen (1983) believes this kind of provision to be mainly of use to carers, whose needs could conceivably be met in other ways. Some innovative homes are built to include a wing for short-stay residents, and to offer adjacent day care.

Day care

This can be provided in day hospitals with an emphasis on further rehabilitation, or by social services, either in residential homes (integrated) or in day centres (segregated). To ensure a normal working day for the transport drivers, half a day of care is more accurately what is provided. For a lonely old person this may be of limited use, as their social circle of people who might visit them at home is not thereby increased, nor does the short day help a working relative with a heavily dependent old person. Yet it does offer a chance to monitor a person's well-being once or twice weekly and can sustain difficult situations in a temporary way to allow fuller assessment and social stimulation.

Neighbourhood initiatives

Social services provision gives increasing emphasis to community social work, with social workers working a small patch in a neighbourhood. The decentralised team gets to know residents in the area well, doing more resource creation, linking old people with those who might for a small payment be able to provide some services. A variety of different schemes have been pioneered around these ideas, notably in Dinnington (Bayley 1984) and in London (Sinclair 1984).

The Kent Community Care scheme (Davies and Challis 1986) has been fully evaluated. It pioneered the idea of giving field social workers financial accountability to buy in and create services, to make up packages that would keep old people at home, provided the total cost did not exceed two-thirds of the cost of residential care.

The concept of key-worker, or care manager, for each old person in need of residential, or the equivalent amount of community, care is now being adopted in many places. Multidisciplinary assessment, a care plan, and periodic reviews, all the elements of child care practice are at last being implemented for old people and endorsed by the Audit Commission (1986). Stronger managerial links with health care are also advocated.

VOLUNTARY SECTOR

The schemes provided by local authorities are replicated by voluntary agencies, taking advantage of their flexibility and independence to pioneer; there are three schemes for fostering old people (Newton 1982). The Meals-on-Wheels service was started in many places by the Womens' Royal Voluntary Service (WRVS) and old peoples' clubs and drop-in centres are organised by small local organisations.

The Crossroads Care Attendant scheme is a voluntary initiative which has spread rapidly. In these schemes the paid care attendant comes in as and when the carer most wants help. The service is free to families (Phillips 1982). The Audit Commission (1986) sees such schemes as the long-term alternative to residential care. For bereaved people there is a nationwide scheme, CRUSE, which might be available to assist newly-bereaved elderly people with counselling and practical help. Age Concern and Help the Aged both act as pressure groups, collate information, provide training facilities, and locally provide particular kinds of day care or regular visiting. Abbeyfield Homes, and others provided by voluntary agencies, offer accommodation with two meals a day and a warden service, a step more than sheltered housing, but less supervision than residential care. (It should be noted in the small print which homes will continue to provide accommodation if the resident becomes ill or disabled, probably needing adaptations to be made.) There are established charities, which offer advice, information, and occasional financial help to those who are in particular difficulties in old age. Taking advantage of voluntary services involves knowing what is available locally and checking out the quality and range of services on offer, matching client and service, once again.

INFORMAL CARE

This represents the essence of community care, meaning that care provided on an informal basis by family, friends and neighbours. As the Audit Commission (1985) pointed out:

> If even a small proportion of those friends and relatives now providing support to elderly people were to 'hand over' their responsibility to the formal sector, the consequences would be serious. Often the carers receive no support from the formal sector, even though saving £3,000 a year for every elderly person looked after, assuming the alternative is local authority residential care.

Levin (1983) in her study of the supporters of confused elderly people, found that those supporters who were most in need of care were receiving least help from the home help service. A series of studies have shown that carers are most likely to be female relatives and that a male carer is more likely to receive a home help, than where there is a woman in the caring role (Equal Opportunities Commission 1982).

Informal care involves both caring for, and caring about the dependent person (Graham 1983). Thus one can well talk of the 'labour of love' for there is much hard work involved, affection, and also more mixed feelings. The point to emphasise here is the 'taken for granted' nature of informal care, which allows costs to be absorbed by the carer, in terms of other activities not pursued, jobs not taken up, pensions not earned, and sometimes physical and mental health injured. The team should take particular note of the pre-retirement single daughter/son prepared to give up job and pension to care for a parent. She/he creates problems for the future. It should not always be assumed that a child cares for a parent. Sometimes the reverse is true.

PRIVATE AND COMMERCIAL SECTOR

There has been an injection of government resources into the commercial sector, by the government's decision in 1982 and 1983 to extend the payment of supplementary benefit board and lodging allowance to private rest home residents, and then to those in private

Table 10.1: Number of residents in private and voluntary homes, people over-65 and younger chronically sick

1984	81,899	
1985	95,841	up 17 per cent
1986	109,607	up 14.4 per cent

Source: Audit Commission (1986)

nursing homes. Those with less than £3,000 capital could claim assistance with fees, provided the local authority could not offer an immediate place in residential accommodation. The figures speak for themselves (Table 10.1). As a result of this increase in the number of residents, in 1985 the rules for payment were tightened. Some of these homes were converted from hotels and guest houses, particularly in coastal areas, with no provision for people not fully able-bodied.

That old age is big business in particularly evident in the sheltered housing market. Some 4,000 to 5,000 units have already been built for private homes, and 15,000 units may be needed annually (Midwinter 1986). The balance between protection and respecting independence of choice is even harder to define in the private and commercial sector. Although many social workers are not comfortable about advising clients on facilities in the private sector, the intermingling of welfare provisions has now become so complex that sometimes clients are better off in the private sector. One difference for admission to private care is the lack of assessment, so that sometimes people do go in who could continue to live at home with more support. Having an alternative kind of care does offer patients and/or their families some kind of choice which should be respected.

FINANCE

Money plays an important part in helping old people sort out the kind of future care that may be most appropriate for them; retirement brings a marked reduction of income. Housing benefit is usually payable for someone on the State pension. Income support is occasionally payable, with an attendance allowance for someone needing help with bodily functions or constant supervision by day and/or by night.

Income in old age reflects that of earlier life; the quality of life may vary enormously. Old women living longest are likely to be among the poorest, as their income diminishes with widowhood; the value of any pension they have declines in value with inflation, and many did not have the opportunity to earn their own pension. Welfare benefits are complicated to work out, and the Citizens' Advice Bureau can offer expert help to social workers on a client's behalf. Although some hospitals have administrative assistants to deal with patients' basic pensions, social workers get tasks such as securing a patients' property in an unlocked flat, dealing with a recalcitrant landlady who wants to evict a tenant while he is in hospital, or paying for kennels for a pet dog.

Decisions about future residential care, requiring careful discussions about income and assets, may be required with the old person and his/her request with relatives. Money is an emotive subject about which people have strong views; residential care must be paid for if there are means; decisions to take up a place are not entirely disinterested, particularly as hospital care is free apart from the deduction in State pension after six weeks. This aspect *might* affect a response to rehabilitation plans, such is the reality of welfare.

Thus the main welfare provisions in the statutory, voluntary, informal and private/commercial sector, have been explored to give some idea of the range available, and of the factors to be borne in mind in helping to plan care with any elderly person. A social worker in rehabilitation work can draw on areas of background knowledge, including the concept of loss, and the ambivalence of dependency which affects both sides in a caring relationship.

PUTTING SOCIAL WORK INTO PRACTICE

Losses in old age

The experience of rehabilitation is probably just one of a number of major physical, emotional and social experiences occurring to an old person. An ageing body brings small decremental losses of eyesight, hearing, memory, and physical activity, before the onset of any major impairment such as a stroke or amputation leads to hospitalisation. The losses in relationships by death, severe illness, or mental infirmity are sometimes felt even more acutely than personal bodily weaknesses, whether it is the death of a spouse, or the grief at the death of siblings and confidantes now being recognised (Wenger 1984; Jerrome 1982). Marris (1986) and Parkes (1986) have helped us to understand the ambivalence of grief, containing within it the shock, immediately followed by numbness, anger/irritability, and then some depression; these earlier griefs could be re-activated with the helplessness following a major physical trauma, and this should be taken into account, if a person is depressed or hard to motivate in rehabilitation.

The prospect of having to give up one's home may cause considerable grief. Tobin and Lieberman (1976) studying people on the waiting list for a nursing home, show that the impact of recognising the inevitability of this step, was the hardest part of the adjustment. Social workers are able to help the rehabilitation team by focusing on the pace of adjustment, and helping the elderly patient through counselling to come to terms with yet more changes, seen in context with their earlier life.

Caring relationships

Parents are used to airing their feelings about children, but feel disloyal airing feelings around old-care, or parent-care. Similarly old people may feel very frustrated at becoming dependent on a younger relative, and either bottle up resentment, or redirect it in some safer direction. Being attached to another when previously there had been considerable independence and autonomy, does create ambivalence (Froggatt 1985). These mixed feelings within a caring relationship reflect the quality of earlier experiences and may contribute to the stress of caring, and being cared for. Thus a social worker needs to get some feel for the family system, as part of his/her contribution to the rehabilitation plan. The possibility that those relationships within the family could come under such stress that violence in the family occurs, should not be overlooked (Cloke 1983).

The attitude of relatives to the impairment, disability and possible handicap of a family member plays a part in a patient's capacity to recover. If, for example, the most important person in the patient's life is distressed by the sight of a badly burned face, recovery and rehabilitation may take longer. A social worker can offer counselling to explore those feelings and help to get through them. Sexual issues should also be considered, for warmth, affection and sexual expression are an important part of personal relationships into advanced old age, yet this is seldom acknowledged (Strean 1983). Advice and support from the rehabilitation team, including the social worker, could assist in this area for a patient or relative seeking clarification of what is medically advisable in the way of resuming intercourse, or of finding other means of sexual expression.

Social work activities

A careful introduction is helpful, to emphasise to the client who the worker is. With an ill or very disabled person two or three short interviews close together may be better, to gain a picture of the problem. A social worker really has to assess the person-in-the-situation for him/herself. Almost no-one is totally isolated; an old man living alone still has neighbours, even if he does not speak to them. There are day-to-day helpers, or carers, all part of the system, affected by the change of health in the patient. These may need to be consulted, if possible with the consent of the patient, only dispensing with this if it is generally agreed that the patient is so mentally infirm that there is an element of protection involved. Building and maintaining trust is an important skill.

Assessment involves being aware of the following interlocking factors: physical health, and mobility; mental state, degree of brain failure, and depression; social circumstances, housing, finance, relatives, neighbours; services received.

Communication with other team members will prevent duplicate assessments and enable tasks to be allocated appropriately. Having weighed up and evaluated these factors, and presented the social report, either verbally or in writing, a care plan will probably be prepared, as suggested. The social worker will continue to have certain tasks.

Two main functions for social workers, of counselling and social care planning, have been defined (Barclay 1982). These are intertwined in most social work activities, including assessment. Unless a patient who has had an amputation is allowed some counselling help, to explore the sense of loss, it could be that the social care planning will not get off the ground, for the future cannot be visualised (see Appendix II).

Discharge from hospital

Ideally, careful social-care planning goes into discharges from hospital. A comprehensive checklist for a full assessment can be found in Marshall (1983). Goldberg and Connelly (1982) spell out the roles that are involved. These are worth looking at in detail.

Mobilisor of resources Having identified the patient's wants, and not merely prescribed an easily available service, a plan for the gaps in the patient's life, on returning home, must be made. What can the person do for him/herself? How long can s/he be left alone? What can relatives and neighbours do? Collating this information may be a team effort, but negotiating for and mobilising the resources is often a social work task. For example, a home help twice a week, Meals-on-Wheels twice a week, and day care once a week might be combined for an old person whose daughter was at work all day.

Co-ordinating and monitoring resources This involves taking particular care to tie-up ends around the time of discharge and making sure the requested services have turned up as required, and are acceptable. Follow-up, by means of a home visit where time permits, can make the difference between a discharge being successful or not. After the tension and encouragement on the ward, a feeling of tiredness, and lassitude often follows at home. At this stage it is easy for an anxious family to do a little too much, and set up a pattern of dependency unnecessarily. It may be that the social work role may not involve *direct counselling* with a patient or relatives, but s/he may be used as a *resource person or consultant* to other rehabilitation team members. Where a hospital social worker has known a patient in hospital s/he will continue to work with that person while out-patient treatment is active. The client/patient will be transferred to a social worker from an area team if ongoing urgent social work support is indicated. Similarly an area social worker may continue to work with a client who has been admitted to hospital, in agreement with the hospital social services team. The choice should be made in the best interests of the client. However, the low priority accorded to elderly people within social service teams means that consistent ongoing social work support may be difficult to offer after discharge from hospital from either source. Voluntary help can sometimes be enlisted to supplement informal care.

Community rehabilitation

It frequently happens that a patient is not referred for social work help while in hospital, but that a referral is made to social services after discharge. For the social worker this will mean working closely with other rehabilitation workers, such as the domiciliary occupational therapist or physiotherapist, and to keep in communication will become more complex. Joint visits are helpful to establish clear lines of work with the family. Family meetings could be considered, including relatives, formal carers (such as home helps) and health-care staff. This is described by Pottle (1984) as part of her psychogeriatric work; a patient needing major rehabilitation might be helped by a similar approach.

There is an awareness within social work that older families too respond to social work intervention. Family therapy in its formal sense may be appropriate, but to include family work in with the other roles can be helpful. For example, one social worker gathered the sons and daughters of a very fierce old lady, into a meeting, so that with support they could each tell her that they could not have her living with them, but would look after her if she went into a home. Until she heard this from all of them at the same time, she would not accept the situation.

Group work is not easy because of a lack of resources, but increasingly there is interest in this kind of work. It could simply be an extension of a 'stroke' class, to allow time for patients to swap experiences. Another group has been tried for patients who are waiting for a place in residential care. Groups for carers are often run, particularly by the Alzheimers' Disease Society.

Reminiscence work using slides, for example *Recall* (Help the Aged 1982) or familiar objects of the past to trigger old memories has become increasingly popular, as a way of stimulating group discussion; groups encouraging patients to write poetry or paint are helpful in encouraging old people to maintain their sense of themselves despite the disruption of hospital life.

CONCLUSION

I hope to have shown the variety of social services that can be available. As often an unqualified assistant is assigned to cover work with elderly people (Black 1983) and to select and negotiate the service required, part of the point of this chapter is to indicate the range of social work skills required, the breadth and depth of work possible with old people and their families. Old people are ourselves 20, 30 or 40 years on. The sense of being many ages at once, of never shedding entirely the youthful inner self, is a feature of old peoples' lives which social workers can respond to and encourage, to help maintain purpose and satisfaction. This kind of skilled and patient work is exemplified in the purposeful and sensitive use of reminiscence (Coleman 1986) as a contribution to rehabilitation work.

This chapter has summarised the main social welfare provisions, and indicated ways in which social workers draw on that knowledge in their work, to individualise a patient and to see the problems of rehabilitation in the context of personal and family circumstances, trying to act as a bridge between that situation and the services that are needed. In this account reference has been made to a number of studies; it is hoped that practitioners from all disciplines will want to read more widely in this field, to help maintain the highest standard of service to elderly people, enabling them to cope with their own lives for as long as possible.

REFERENCES

Age Concern (1986) *The Law and Vulnerable Elderly People.* Age Concern, Mitcham

Allen, I. (1983) *Short-Stay Residential Care for the Elderly.* Policy Studies Institute, London

Audit Commission (1985) *Managing Social Services for the Elderly More Effectively.* HMSO, London
—— (1986) *Making a Reality of Community Care.* HMSO, London, Table D-1, 124

Barclay, P. (1982) *Social Workers, Their Role and Tasks.* National Institute of Social Work, (Bedford Square Press), London

Bayley, M. (1984) *Neighbourhood Services Project — Dinnington Papers.* University of Sheffield, Department of Sociology, Sheffield

Black, J. (1983) *Social Work in Context.* Tavistock Publications, London

Bury, M.R. (1979) Disablement in Society. *International Journal of Rehabilitation Research, 2,* 1, 34–40

Cloke, C. (1983) *Old Age Abuse in the Domestic Setting.* Age Concern, Mitcham

Coleman, P. (1986) *Ageing and Reminiscence Processes.* Wiley, Chichester

Davies, B. and Challis, D. (1986) *Matching Resources to Needs in Community Care.* Gower, Aldershot

Equal Opportunities Commission (1982) *Caring for the Elderly and Handicapped.* HMSO, London

Froggatt, A. (1985) Adult Children. Paper presented at British Society of

Gerontology Conference, University of Keele, Hull

Glendinning, F. (1982) *Care in the Community: Recent Research and Development*. University of Keele, Beth Johnson Foundation with Department of Adult Education and Age Concern

Goldberg, E.M. and Connelly, N. (1982) *The Effectiveness of Social Care of the Elderly*. Heinemann Educational, London

Graham, H. (1983) Caring: A Labour of Love. In J. Finch and D. Groves, *A Labour of Love*. Routledge & Kegan Paul, London

Help the Aged (1982) *Recall*. Help the Aged, London

Jerrome, D. (1982) Men Women and Friendship in Old Age. Unpublished paper presented at British Society of Gerontology Conference, University of Keele, Hull

Latto, S. (1982) Managing the Care System. In F. Glendinning, *op. cit.*

Levin, E. (1983) *The Supporters of Confused Elderly People at Home*. National Institute of Social Work, London

Levin, E. Sinclair, I. and Gorbach, P. (1985) The effectiveness of the home help service with confused old people and their families. *Research Policy and Planning*, *3*, 2, 1–7

Marris, P. (1986) *Loss and Change*. Routledge & Kegan Paul, London

Marshall, M. (1983) *Social Work with Elderly People*. British Association of Social Work, with Macmillan, Basingstoke

Midwinter, E. (1986) *Caring for Cash*. Centre for Policy on Ageing, London

Newton, S. (1982) A Short Term Boarding Out Scheme for the Elderly. In F. Glendenning, *op. cit.*

Norman, A. (1985) *Triple Jeopardy*. Centre for Policy on Ageing, London

Parker, G. (1985) *With Due Care and Attention*. Family Policy Studies Centre, London

Parkes, C.M. (1986) *Bereavement: Studies of Grief in Adult Life*. Penguin Books, Harmondsworth with Tavistock, London

Phillips, D. (1982) The Crossroads Care Attendant Scheme. In F. Glendinning, *op. cit.*

Phillipson, C. and Walker, A. (1986) *Ageing and Social Policy*. Gower, Aldershot

Pottle, S. (1984) Developing a network-oriented service for elderly people. In A. Treacher and J. Carpenter, *Using Family Therapy*. Blackwell, Oxford

Sinclair, I. (1984) *Networks Project: A Study of Informal Care, Services and Social Work for Elderly Clients Living Alone*. National Institute of Social Work Research Unit, London

Strean, H. (1983) *The Sexual Dimension*. The Free Press, New York

Tinker, A. (1981) *The Elderly in Modern Society*. Longman, London

Tobin, S. and Lieberman, M.A. (1976) *The Last Refuge*. Jossey-Bass, San Francisco

Ware, P. (1983) *Boarding Out/Fostering of Elderly People in the United Kingdom*. Unpublished M.Phil. University of Bradford, Bradford

Wenger, C. (1984) *The Supportive Network*. George Allen & Unwin, London

Willcocks, D. (1986) Residential Care. In C. Phillipson and A. Walker, *op. cit.*

11

Home Assessment

Penelope Fenn Clark and Katherine Coombes

Most of the studies which have been published in the English-language journals, on functional assessment, while specific to particular age groups or diagnoses, have not limited themselves solely to the patient's own home. The original assessment is more often undertaken in the hospital, for this is where the patient and the multidisciplinary team are first introduced to one another (Rossman 1983). But some will be undertaken by community staff where the patient has not needed hospitalisation (see Chapters 12 and 13). Some hospital- or clinic-based ADL (Activities of Daily Living) trials, while mentioning rehabilitation and discharge, never make reference to the patients' homes at all, yet it is at home that these activities, or the lack of them, will be most crucial to the patient's independence. So it is the home itself which may be the key factor in determining whether the tested ADL will be continued after discharge, and which may be in as urgent need of attention as the patient (Howell 1986; Rossman 1983).

For the purposes of this chapter the home assessment will be defined as a visit with a patient to his or her home, or to the patient already at home, by a member or members of the multidisciplinary team in order to assess the patient's level of safe independence at home, for mobility and ADL, and to recommend input or action to achieve optimum quality of life with appropriate support and services. A visit without the patient is also possible and often valuable early in the admission.

Once a hospitalised patient has recovered sufficient functional independence for the eventual discharge to become a feasible aim, it will be appropriate for the rehabilitation efforts of the team to be directed towards the discharge destination. It is commonplace to assume that the patient will eventually return to the place whence he came — his 'home'. This may not prove to be possible or even desirable, but it is the starting point for the discharge plans. If discharge to other accommodation (e.g. Part III, sheltered or nursing home) is planned, a visit to ensure facilities and furniture are adequate for the patient will not only benefit the patient but provide liaison between hospital and community. When a patient is attending out-patient or day care facility, it is helpful and appropriate for the home assessment to be undertaken fairly soon, in order to determine the goals of rehabilitation treatment. Thus, the timing of the visit — or perhaps the need for more than one home assessment — will vary according to the patient's ability and prognosis, and according to the type of accommodation occupied before the current episode.

The patient will have been assessed by the team in hospital and the home assessment will compare findings and test abilities in the 'real' situation, aiming to ensure the patients' maximum independence and safety in their dwelling. In the present economic climate, in pressurised health districts, there may be a diversity of hidden aims cherished by different members of the multidisciplinary team, such as to achieve higher turnover of beds, to reduce admission rates, to minimise referral to out-patient departments.

The patient's own desires may prove somewhat high-flown compared with the realities of the case, and however much laudable effort is expended in securing maximal quality of life for those in our care, it is also part of the role of home assessor to help the patient to come to terms creatively with the diminishment which disability heralds. It may not be time wasted, during a home assessment, to help a severely disabled patient up stairs that she will probably never climb again, to say 'Goodbye', to direct which furniture she would like brought downstairs for a projected bed-sitting room, or even just to show the bed where her 13 children were born. 'Time remember'd is grief forgotten' (Swinburne 1865).

It may require patience, persuasion and perseverance to reconcile a keen gardener after a severe stroke, to the fact that the steps down from the back-door are an overwhelming non-negotiable hazard; only by allowing the patient to attempt this without help, catching him as he begins to fall, may it be possible to let the sad truth sink home. The thought of returning home to watch a prized garden run wild is a certain recipe for depression and social work intervention may enable a local flat dweller to take it on as a hobby or part of a 'paid neighbour' scheme if desired by the owner (Chambers 1986).

Acceptance requires time (Kübler-Ross 1970), and a tactful interval for grief should be allowed before proffering suggestions of window boxes, potted plants or goldfish. Such sensitivity is even more important when the reason for the assessment is to make it obvious to all concerned that a return to life at home is barely possible at all.

To include an assessment of the patient's hobbies and recreational interests at home, and to plan ways in which these can be resumed, will enhance the motivation of the patient towards successful discharge.

COMPOSITION OF THE VISITING TEAM

Where a team of hospital personnel is dealing with the patient, each or any one of them may decide that a home assessment is needed, because of particular difficulties the patient has been found to have in the hospital setting, and where suggestions or methods of dealing with them there may not be applicable at home. When the multidisciplinary team meets, be it ward round, case conference or team discussion, the members broach the subject and discuss the indications for carrying out a home assessment. For example, once it has become apparent to the physiotherapy staff that the patient will probably not be able to walk safely alone, it is sensible to ensure that any walking aid or wheelchair will fit in and between the room(s) that he will occupy at home; or if a patient previously capable of stairclimbing becomes confined to one level, an early visit to the home will reveal whether this is feasible, with aids and adaptations or whether rehousing is the only option. Much staff time and effort may otherwise be directed towards ends which prove at the last minute to be unattainable due to the structure and layout of the home itself.

The decision as to who will carry out the visit is made by self-election and the team's concurrence. The occupational therapist will most likely be the key home assessor, with perhaps the physiotherapist where problems hinge on mobility, or the speech therapist where dysphasia is the major problem, or social worker where social issues are paramount. Whichever member of the team has the specific skills and experience relevant to the patient's needs should be involved.

Whoever carries out the home assessment will bear in mind the necessity of onward referral of other problems which may be revealed, to the appropriate staff or organisation. They will be the eyes and ears of the whole team. The perception of the staff who carry out the visit (which profession and what level of experience) may influence what is found. It is often helpful for all concerned for a new member of the team to visit with a more experienced member, not necessarily of the same discipline. Students of all disciplines gain valuable insight into the living conditions — good or bad — of old people and should be included whenever possible, with the patient's agreement.

PREPARATION

The home assessment cannot be made without preliminary ground-work. Familiarity with the patient, the medical notes, results of any other assessments already made, the present level of functional ability, state of motivation, and the course of progress in rehabilita-tion to date, are basic prerequisites. Diagnosis and prognosis may reflect the dependency level which may be anticipated, and whether short- or long-term incapacity should be planned for (Kramer *et al.* 1985). To return a patient to a situation which is just about manageable on good days will cause hardship, suffering and disap-pointment for the patient, and may provoke re-admission. In some cases, especially where resources are planned so that the patient's rehabilitation will be continued in and from the home (Jarnlo *et al.* 1984), there may be certain areas of improvement on discharge, but in general a progressive diminishment must be catered for (Sheikh *et al.* 1979; Mahoney and Barthel 1965; Haworth and Hollings 1979).

If possible, a meeting with those who form part of the support network in the community (relatives, friends, statutory social or health services representatives) will reveal whether it would be helpful for them to be present at the home assessment too. They might usefully demonstrate previous difficulties or even the precipitating cause of admission, but hospital staff must be sensitive to resistance from those who have been caring successfully for years and may resent a one-off 'intrusion'. The sheer numbers of people must be limited so as not to overwhelm the patient or crowd the home, or to raise the cost of staff time, but a minimum of two, especially on a visit to an unavoidably empty home to deter accusations of theft, and as physical support when so-called 'no-go'

187

areas must be visited.

The patient's address will supply an indication of the neighbourhood, proximity of local amenities, shops, access and transport. The level of vandalism in the area will probably be obvious and may not only affect the older person going out, but also the availability of door-to-door services. The patient's type of housing will have been ascertained during the course of thorough documentation on admission or original assessment, with such details as the number of floors, presence, reliability or absence of a lift, distance between the front door and the nearest set-down point. To take a wheelchair may avoid exhausting the patient before the assessment even begins.

The elderly in the United Kingdom tend to occupy poorer housing stock with fewer domestic amenities than average households (Fox 1981) and to remain static within upwardly mobile populations, having neither energy, enthusiasm, nor often, finances to press for maintenance and repair of the property they live in. Elderly owner-occupiers are often left in large family homes, leading to neglect of house (and garden). Failure of the ability to care for one's home is listed by Barber (1984) as one of the functional incapacities which, with mobility and self-care loss, lead to dependency. Some defects may be noted and remedied as a consequence of a period of hospitalisation. Even when rehousing is recommended many people will still chose 'home' as their ideal place to be, and it cannot be part of the rehabilitation team's remit radically to alter more than those factors which will effect a safe discharge. There is a largely unfulfilled role for team members to play in advising people, in advance of disability, on suitable housing, furniture, etc. (Griffiths 1973).

Occasionally, such appalling conditions are found that a dwelling may be unfit for human habitation. If the visitors find evidence of vermin, a grossly unsafe building, extensive damp, rot or other fundamental health hazards, the matter must be referred immediately, usually through the social work department, for action by social services, the public health department of the local council or other relevant body.

Before the home assessment the staff concerned will do well to discover the patient's and main carers' expectations and to explain the purpose of the visit. Between the poles of sheer survival and full self-determination lie many levels of safe coping, requiring many levels of outside help. Relief of family stress and neighbourly concern, availability of statutory provisions and reduction of emergency calls, will all bear on the eventual scheme of care, aids and adaptations recommended (Sanford 1975). The necessary skills for maximum independence and safety may need rehearsal at home, e.g. cooking in the patient's own kitchen if the patient has a history of malnutrition, or getting up from the floor or raising the alarm if there is a history of falls.

The patient demonstrates abilities as much to him/herself as to the visiting staff, thus counteracting the pessimistic and negative effects of the process of illness, emergency and admission to hospital. It is, therefore, encouraging for the patient to be told about the proposed visit at an early stage, to motivate further rehabilitative efforts.

PLANNING THE VISIT

When the team has decided on the date, time and whom to depute, the visit should be logged in the appropriate diary. One of the team sets aside time to tell the patient, explain the procedure and determine access to the property. There may be people to contact in advance: family at home, a key-holder neighbour, the warden of sheltered accommodation, and community staff as relevant.

It is vital to emphasise to the patient that this homecoming is not permanent, and not a kind of test or 'exam', but is to solve problems in advance. As the key person, (s)he does not have to prove him/herself, but may safely share problems and concerns with the staff. Some patients, remembering disorganisation or questionable cleanliness left behind upon hurried admission, are afraid of staff misjudgment, or become aware of their role as host(ess) and are reluctant to allow anyone to see the home before they have a chance to tidy up. (Readers may like to consider their own reaction to visitors viewing their home as they left it this morning!) Patients' questions and fears should be met with understanding and sensitivity by someone who has established a rapport already. Health-care personnel on home visits yet remain essentially as guests in the patient's home.

Some patients imagine they must pay for or arrange the journey themselves; while explaining travel arrangements staff can ask about motion sickness problems and request appropriate medication as necessary. Ensure that the patient is sufficiently agile to get into the car, and that the car itself is of a suitable make, model and size to accommodate any particular disability (e.g, arthrodesed knee) and to carry equipment which may be needed on the assessment or delivered to the home (Squires 1984). Most hospitals have established straightforward transport procedures, taxicab contracts, League of Friends drivers' rosters or informal volunteers, and one needs to follow the agreed practice. In health districts where staff use their own cars, a block insurance policy is taken out by the Authority in respect of such cars, and it is vital to inform the relevant administrators of the necessary vehicle and driver details.

Where the front door of the home can only be reached by stairs which a patient cannot climb, a two-man ambulance must be ordered for the patient and escort. The ambulance personnel will be responsible for carrying the patient from the vehicle to the home, for which they are both trained and covered by insurance, while the rehabilitation staff attend to equipment and aids they need to bring.

It is vital to make arrangements for return to the hospital at the same time as planning the outward journey, and to check these with the driver before leaving the hospital. It is safer to postpone the assessment than to risk being stranded with the patient at home, possibly far from the nearest telephone. This eventuality would at least highlight for the team the patient's potential danger from isolation!

An updated map with the route ready planned, and the key to the property are essential prerequisites — the latter may seem obvious but is not an unknown omission!

There will be other things to take on a home assessment as well as those already mentioned. If home visits are carried out frequently it is convenient to assemble some of the standard items in a holdall. A home visit holdall content checklist might read:

- address of the patient
- road map
- money — for emergency expenditure
- phonecard
- telephone numbers — hospital and patient's own doctor
- stationery — for ticklists, sketches, measurement jottings, etc.
- measuring tape or steel rule
- marking tabs — self-adhesive, to mark positions of grabrails, etc.
- ingredients — for kitchen assessment
- cameras — and photography consent forms

— medications — if unavoidably due during visit
— receptacle — (polythene bag and tissues) in case of travel sickness
— incontinence pads
— 'refusal to return to hospital' form (= 'self-discharge')

Remember a routine pre-embarkation trip to the toilet, and possibly restriction of fluids beforehand. If incontinence is anticipated, padded pants (or even temporary catheterisation) may be indicated.

The patient should be suitably clad and shod for the weather, with extra clothing even if not required *en route*, as the patient will be acclimatised to high ward temperatures. A house temporarily unoccupied and unheated may be visited earlier by a friend or neighbour, though finances may be threatened by having to warm the house for the short time it will be required.

On the journey the visitor(s) will note the situation of the home in its neighbourhood and environs (the position of a dwelling unit in a multiple-occupancy building, or the appearance, size and condition of house and garden, etc.), the immediate access and problems the patient has in traversing uneven ground, slopes, steps, etc. before reaching the front door. The patient should rely on such help as would normally be available from rails, walking aid or a supportive companion preferably present in person, to use the opportunity for observation and instruction (or even for the staff to gain useful experience of non-professionals' knacks and expertise). Never underestimate the amount of help two frail people can exchange very safely because of their intimate knowledge and mutual confidence.

ASSESSMENT

The assessment is in two parts: firstly to ascertain the present situation (from the observation of which, the problems can be listed), and secondly to determine what should be done to enable the patient to live here safely with maximum functional independence.

Observations of the patient's abilities should include all areas which will be used, and access and mobility in and between relevant rooms. If possible, and with the patient's agreement, minor recommendations should be fulfilled at the time, and the patient encouraged to try out the new circumstances, e.g. raised toilet seat, half-step, re-positioning of table.

Though it may be tempting to reorganise a household completely, in the interests of safety, it may prove less safe to move things because an older person's proprioceptive sense of their position, neuronally reinforced over the years, will not accommodate readily, and patients with sensory, especially visual, deficit may become downright confused. One of the major skills of the home assessor is to elicit from the family or the patient what changes could be helpful. This way the change is already 'sold' and the initiative is life-enhancing. Autocratic dogmatic manners should be avoided by the therapists lest the patient refuse help, which if hinted at tactfully, might have been accepted. Even if the patient is receptive, never make wild claims of possible changes or help available. Note needs and requests, and report accordingly.

Underlying the particular and general aims of any one assessment, broad categories of observations are made, some in particular rooms, some relevant throughout the home:

— access and mobility
— structural soundness
— flooring (type and covering)
— lighting — intensities and switch types
— accessibility of power points and switches
— heating methods — room and water
— cooking facilities
— fuel sources
— hygiene and washing facilities
— communication with the outside world
— alarm and support systems where independence falls short

A discussion of these, what might be found, and suggestions of ways of dealing with some of the problems will lead to a consideration of methods of reporting back to the multidisciplinary team.

Access and mobility

The builder's target market is young, fit healthy people, agile, able and strong. Having reached the accommodations, elderly people meet their first obstacle at the front door. The doorstep may be too high and neither broad enough to stand on, nor narrow enough to step over. The height and width of the door-sill and any protruding ledges will be noted. Doormats do not provide firm standing and may slide on the underlying floor covering. The key may be stiff to turn, the front door difficult to open, and once open, may swing shut again threatening insecure balance. The patient may be tempted to leave it ajar for visitors rather than face repeated trips to answer the bell (a dangerous practice these days, which sufficient duplicate keys for frequent callers can remedy). A raised box or shelf at the front door will prevent the patient (and the milkman!) having to bend to retrieve bottles. While letter baskets inside the door prevent mail falling to the floor, they can obstruct access through the doorway.

A walking frame may prove more of an encumbrance than a help, where there are steps or stairs, and it may be preferable to have grab-rails or bannisters fixed at the point of difficulty, and issue extra frames for use on the upper levels. Anticipated improvement in the patient's strength and range of movement would reduce the effort involved, so careful measurement of the tread depth, riser height and stair nosing dimensions will enable the patient and the rehabilitation team to work to a known target. The assessors and the patient must decide whether it is necessary to have to climb (flights of) stairs at all, or if the living accommodation can be rearranged on one level. If the patient admits that the stairs are all but over-whelming the team will have a plan of action to suggest.

The space occupied by any mobility aid needs consideration. The width and length of a walking frame, and where it will be parked when not in use, yet still within reach of the patient, must be worked out with its user and other inhabitants. The turning circle and clearance required for a wheelchair must be tested out in practice.

The speed at which the patient can move safely about the home should be noted and, if excessively slow, care staff calling in future may be warned not to expect an instant answer to their knock. The incidence of deafness in the community is probably twice that reported (Herbst and Humphrey 1980), so the home assessment provides an excellent opportunity to test whether the patient can hear the knocker or doorbell while listening to the radio or television. Louder bells, a different pitch or tone quality could be recom-mended, or a flashing light. Referral to the hospital audiology department may be appropriate.

Structure

A home may be owned by its occupier or by one of a wide range of public or private agencies, so any recommended alteration or addition to the permanent structure of the building must be cleared with the appropriate body; from the re-hanging of a door, or fixing of a wall hand-rail to complement the bannisters (private landlords might refuse permission), to the building of an extension for a downstairs toilet (owner-occupiers need borough council planning permission and must conform to local bye-laws). The foreseeable difficulties may actually limit or dictate the extent of structural alterations, especially where a large expenditure would be incurred. Richer patients may ask for advice on how to engage the necessary labour; impecunious patients may need someone to negotiate with landlords on their behalf. While it is desirable for the therapist to be consulted about physical details, distances and measurements and appropriate fixtures, referral should be made to the patient's social worker for help with grants, permission and contractors, unless a competent and willing relative is prepared to. The same applies to the problems that arise when the patient cannot go home until the fixtures are in place, but the workmen cannot go into the home until there is someone there!

Before suggesting any fixed aids, account should be taken of the fixing points. Plaster-board walls will not necessarily take the installation of a firm grab-rail without reinforcement. Taps and pipes may not be firm enough for a tap-anchored bath-rail. An extra power socket may not be possible where the ring-main already has its full load.

Security

The balance between allowing access to the welcome visitor and the barring of entry to the unwanted intruder in any home is problematic, and for the elderly the problems are compounded. Locks and catches may be stiff or worn, loose or ineffective; and bolts are situated at the top and bottom of doors, both positions difficult for those with limited ability to reach and bend. Failing vision may render security spy-holes useless. The elderly may not have heard or grasped the import of frequent media warnings never to open the door to an unexpected, unidentified caller, or to be suspicious of self-styled public utilities officers, meter-readers, etc. who fail to produce credentials or to wear uniform. A door chain is a simple, cheap and easily-installed device, but, unless it incorporates a padlock, will prevent authorised entry by known key-holders when the person within cannot release it. A note on the inside of the door reminding the occupier not to let strangers in may help.

Windows should be openable by the inhabitant(s) for desired ventilation in hot weather, but are notorious points of entry for housebreakers. If security is in doubt, the Crime Prevention Officer of the local police station can be commended to the householder as a source of advice.

Flooring

The very first and most important question to ask about the floor is: 'is there one?' With nearly one-third of Britain's housing stock having been built prior to 1914 (Marshall 1987), and many properties seriously deteriorated, it is a false assumption that every home has wall-to-wall flooring! People become accustomed to avoiding their known household hazards, and may automatically avoid treading on the weak spots, until failing balance and slower righting reflexes put them at the double risk not only of falling, but of falling through.

The assessor will aim to achieve for the patient a floor which is level and smooth. The sheer structure and age of some housing renders this a counsel of perfection. Carpets cover a multitude of horrors. Without trying to become structural surveyors, the visiting staff may be able to suggest to the owner, landlord or relevant council housing department, that structural maintenance is a wise investment, and cannot reduce the value of the property, even if they are reluctant to undertake repairs for the sake of the inhabitant in question.

The patient or family should be encouraged and persuaded to remove slip-mats (so rightly named), despite the reasonable explanation for their presence. Overlapping edges of carpet, linoleum or vinyl floor coverings should be marked and unsafe sections referred to the relevant department. Perhaps white stripping or paint can be used at any change in height of flooring. If you cannot win, at least try and lose with safety still paramount.

Lighting

The assessors should bear in mind that the lighting levels indoors will vary considerably with the time of day and season of the year.

Assessments carried out on a summer morning should also include a consideration of how the patient will see to get to the toilet in the middle of the night or on a late afternoon in December. Bulbs of a higher wattage may be needed especially in passages, hallways, over stairs and steps, and switches need to be situated so that an area can be illuminated remotely before the patient has to enter it.

The acquisition of a bedside torch or fluorescent 'glow-worm' plug can overcome the absence of a bedside lamp, though its presence can cause alternative problems, as the elderly eye requires more time to accommodate to brilliance. It should be remembered that to an old person a 'night-light' is synonymous with a 'candle' so careful choice of words will avoid this hazard. The human eye requires four times as much light to see as well at the age of 50 as it did at 20, so many elderly people will already have made their own arrangements for the siting of light fixtures long before they become our patients.

The assessor may need to note types of switches which cause difficulties. A background knowledge of the available range of types on the market will enable suitable recommendations to be made, selecting from rocker-switch, tab, pull-cord, torpedo switch or press-button according to disability. Self-triggering 'welcome light' sensors may be useful in hallways.

The visually handicapped may benefit from the use of alternative light sources, e.g. fluorescent tubes, tinted bulbs. If vision is a key problem at home, referral to the ophthalmic department of the hospital can yield useful advice, and the patient be enabled to receive the benefits of becoming registered as partially sighted. Some poor lighting is caused simply because the patient cannot reach to change the light bulb, and nobody has called to whom the request could be made. It should not be assumed that electricity is laid on. A number of homes in the United Kingdom still (1988) have gas lighting.

Power and fuel sources

Power sockets in the United Kingdom are often sited close to floor level. While this reduces the hazard of trailing leads, it renders switches and plugs inaccessible to those with bending or reaching difficulties (but puts them within easy reach of babies and toddlers!). Electrical appliances and wiring may appear dangerously old and worn, and a check by the local electricity board may be recommended, although unfortunately, recommendations cannot be enforced, nor can money always be found to fund replacements. Simple home-made devices, such as a rubber thimble on the end of a dowelling stick to flick switches on and off are cheap and instant remedies. Electric plugs with handles for easy withdrawal cost only about half as much again as ordinary plugs. (The electricity board will always be willing to advise disabled people on specific equipment for their needs and disabilities.)

Where electricity is not the main fuel source, other problems may arise. Self-ignition gas-taps within easy reach are ideal, but where absent, safe ways of applying the lighted match to the gas jet often at ground level, soon after turning on the supply, must be evolved if the patient is to avoid becoming a potential explosion hazard. Coin-box meters may be in impossibly dangerous or difficult positions for the elderly to reach, but can be changed on request, or neighbours and home helps alerted to the necessity of topping up the meter at intervals.

Solid fuel fires and cookers require the carrying of often heavy loads of fuel inbound and ashes outbound. Securing ventilation for open and closed combustion fires while avoiding draughts, arranging for flue maintenance and chimney sweeping may tax the stamina of those with diminished exercise tolerance, leading to neglect of safety measures. Fire-guards should always be used with open (and perhaps other) fires. Old style paraffin heaters need regular and careful maintenance for safety, and even the modern safety models with automatic extinguishers in case of overturning, still have to be filled, heavy cans have to be carried, and accurate pouring for refilling is vital. A wide-mouthed funnel and a stool or box on which to rest the can while pouring may aid patients with weakness or tremor.

The type of heating and the patient's ability to use it should be tested even on a summer visit: winter will come. The coldest rooms in a house without central heating are often the toilet (bathroom) and the bedroom, precisely where undressing heightens susceptibility to loss of body heat and onset of hypothermia. The risk of hypothermia in countries with cold winters is of great public concern — but usually only during the winter. Dressing and undressing, if slow risky procedures in themselves, should take place in the warm if possible. The assessor should detect any reluctance to use the heating available, where financial hardship is the likely cause, as the risk of hypothermia increases with low income (Jordan 1978). If present heating methods are ineffective perhaps replacement (e.g. of an electric bar heater by a fan-heater) would achieve better space heating for the same expenditure.

The exceptionally cold winter of 1987 in the United Kingdom gave rise to a plethora of public advice on ways of keeping warm, including re-statements of standing invitations to the elderly and ill to apply to their social security offices for help in cash or kind. If patients in need have not already done so, they may be glad of the help or prompting of a social worker.

Cooking facilities

If the home has been unoccupied and unattended since the day of the patient's admission to hospital, the visitors will have to be prepared for a little housework themselves, to see to any minor clearing up, but in the case of major cleaning being needed, it may be necessary to postpone this part of the assessment until, through the social worker, the 'dirty squad' department of the home help service can be called on to overhaul the cleanliness of the kitchen or any other room(s) in which it may be needed.

The assessment carried out in the occupational therapy department kitchen in hospital will have revealed possible problems to be reviewed at home, as performance is invariably compromised in an unfamiliar set-up. At minimum, the preparation of a cup of tea, buttered toast, and a boiled egg will demonstrate a representative range of necessary skills, and other abilities required (e.g. opening tins, taking hot dishes from the oven, reaching the cupboards, carrying utensils across the kitchen, using the refrigerator) may be performed too. Here, as throughout the home, difficulties will be recognised by the visitors or expressed by the patient, remedies sought and suggested, or notes taken for action later.

Hygiene and washing facilities

The ability to keep oneself and one's environment clean is fundamental to human dignity and self-respect, yet requires an agility and stamina which become progressively more difficult with increasing age (Lundgren-Lindquist et al. 1983). The layout of the plumbing itself may be the cause of the difficulties, and will need a critical examination with a view to possible helpful changes.

The assessors should note the position and accessibility of washbasins, sinks and bathrooms, and the patient's ability to turn the taps. The toilet, colloquially 'the smallest room' is often exactly that in reality and may not be wide enough to admit a walking-frame or wheelchair, though aided-ambulant patients may be able to use handholds to reach the toilet. Sometimes multiple sideways transfers via chairs and laundry-box stools will enable a patient to get there but this is a tiring regime, and the furniture involved may obstruct other family members. The seat may be too low, and a raised toilet seat or frame incorporating a raise may be needed. Toilet paper and the flushing chain or handle should be within reach. Where other methods fail, there is an inaccessible outside toilet, or getting there at night is a particularly hazardous undertaking for the patient, a commode may have to be obtained. Foresight must be exercised in planning for its emptying, although modern 'camping' toilets now make this a weekly rather than a daily event.

Where there is an accessible bathroom and the patient wishes to use the bath, the safety of getting in and out will need to be checked, and bath-boards, rails, nonslip mats, etc. recommended as appropriate. A bath-attendant may be available if the patient is deemed to be at high risk when attempting to bath alone. The installation of a shower may be a preferable alternative.

Water-heating methods vary considerably, often linked to room or house heating system. Where there is no plumbed hot water and the patient has to boil in on the stove, the safety of this method should be reviewed, especially the carrying of hot vessels from the stove to wherever the hot water will be used.

The general level of hygiene and cleanliness throughout the dwelling, and primarily in connection with food preparation and consumption, will be assessed along with rehearsal of the patient's activities in these quarters.

Furniture

The assessors should note the stability, type, solidity and height of all relevant furniture and suggest that the patient demonstrates the use of the items habitually in use, checking on the points which cause difficulty or appear unsafe. Furniture on wheels or casters, which the patient uses for stability, are best blocked by caster-coasters. Stiff handles or hinges may need oiling, knob-handles may need replacement by lever types or relocation at different heights, latches may not catch properly. Chests of drawers may not open easily, and wardrobe doors may not stay open, both endangering precarious balance. Humans are naturally acquisitive, so an average elderly person's home is likely to become crowded. A few extra items may be useful as handholds, and strategically placed chairs on the level and on landings may enable the severely dyspnoeic patient to rest sufficiently to move about. Chairfast or ambulant, the patient should demonstrate safe mobility to the assessors, and be encouraged to discard unnecessary, obstructive or dangerous furniture.

Chairs

It should be possible to select from the range of types of chairs already in the home, chairs to suit the needs and usage of the individual patient. Aim for firmness, a sound back support, a design which allows the hips, knees and ankles of the sitter to rest at right-angles and for the patient to be able to rise from sitting (with nothing to block the feet from being drawn back beneath the body's centre of gravity). Demonstration of the inability to rise from a chair may help to persuade its owner to replace it. The height can be raised, most safely with linked blocks which will move as a unit with the chair. Cushions can compensate for insufficient height or too long a seat. Chair arms should be at the right height to provide rest for the forearms, and firm enough and far enough forward to assist rising. If the household has no suitable chair, one which fits the occupant should be provided. If it is known that a person will sleep in the chair at night, arrange the best possible position and provide an easily moveable footrest of the correct height — recliner chairs have proved useful for this — the important point to make is that the leg level raises high enough to prevent postural oedema.

Wheelchair users wishing to transfer to other chairs should be monitored for transfer safety with brakes *on*, and heights and stability adjusted.

Tables

They should be steady and at the correct height for their usage. There should be space beneath for the knees of wheelchair users, perhaps using an alternative pair of 'desk arms' to enable the patient to sit closer to the table. It may be possible to raise a table slightly with firm fixed blocks, but this can make the surface too high for comfort.

Bed

The ideal here is for a steady bed with a firm, level mattress at the right height for transfers or getting in and out, with sufficient bedclothes and pillows. Low beds can be raised with bed-blocks which should be firmly fixed, but this is not ideal as moving the bed loses the blocks. A second firm mattress or the addition of neatly folded layers of spare bedding give the same result. A board can support a spongy mattress and obscure the effects of broken bed-springs. Therapists are sometimes asked to raise one end of the bed for medical effect, but the use of bed-blocks for this will destroy the balance of many beds, causing jack-knife and shearing stresses at the junction of the frame with the headboard or footboard. Unless the bed is a divan type it will be safer to place wedges or spare bedding under the mattress. Divan beds cause problems by preventing the person's feet from getting far enough back for safe standing transfers.

The proximity of a firm chair or chair-type commode for lower limb amputees may be a vital part of dressing independence. A double bed now occupied by one person may make getting in and out more difficult but sensitivity should be used when suggesting a replacement. The position of the bed within the room must also be assessed for the patient's disability (e.g. a left hemiplegic will be safer getting in towards his affected side so that a fall will only be onto the bed).

It is not wise to assume that all people 'go to bed' at night. Some elderly people, worried that they are unable to get to the toilet quickly enough, have for some time slept in a chair and actually disposed of their bed. Search for a non-existent 'bedroom' can be most disorientating for the assessors!

Communication systems

The danger of an elderly housebound person becoming isolated and having no way to raise the alarm in a crisis should be borne in mind by the visiting team.

It has been suggested by Barker and Bury (1978) that the state of being housebound is itself linked to mortality, and in their Spaulding Rehabilitation Hospital House Visit Evaluation Form, Rosenblatt *et al.* (1986) take it as normative that all patients be rated for their ability to escape from the house in emergency. Communication with the outside world is a two-way process, initiated either from other people contacting the patient or from the patient's own initiative. The informal social network may be adequate for maintaining checks on both the property and the health of the person at risk. Other family members living with the patient will be in a position to call for appropriate assistance when required, unless both members of an elderly couple become incapacitated simultaneously.

Old people living alone are deemed to be at risk solely because of having nobody at home with them (Macmillan 1960), and special provisions must be made to enable them to make outside contacts. A basic intervention would be the installation of a telephone (funding may be available in some cases through the social worker) with at least the ability to dial or trigger a 999 call. The accessibility of a telephone can be enhanced by the addition of a second machine, alternative sockets or cordless models. A handy and clearly legible list of emergency numbers is useful. (Recent advances in British Telecom's provisions for specific handicaps are outlined in their publication *Action for disabled customers* which is sent free of charge to subscribers upon request.)

A telephone is often a prerequisite for some of the alarm systems which may be provided by local social services, but provision for these is patchy, and varies from borough to borough. Similarly, a variety of private organisations run telephone-linked body-worn alert-button systems, but availability is not uniform throughout the United Kingdom. Interesting developments in the use of Citizens Band (CB) radio with older people are described by Hill-Tout (undated). A display of communication systems is situated at the Disabled Living Foundation along with other items enhancing the life of disabled people.

The assessors can enquire whether neighbours would hear or respond to a shout or a knock on the wall. Some local Age Concern, 'Good Neighbours', 'Crossroads' or similar schemes furnish their elderly residents with 'HELP' cards to display in the window for urgent assistance (unfortunately also visible to those tempted to take advantage of vulnerability). Baby-care alarm systems can easily be adopted for use by the elderly who live close enough to their main carer.

METHODOLOGY AND REPORTS

From the above outline it can be seen that the range of possible problems which may confront the patient and the visiting assessment team is very wide. Standard local tick-lists or check-points prevent serious omissions, and perhaps indicate a customary format for the report. An accurate if scribbled note made at the time on site is much more valuable than memory-dependent guesses. One suggested method of ensuring that every activity is tested is to take the patient through the day's movements, from getting out of bed, dressing, washing, grooming, etc. (Trombly and Scott 1977) or it may be more convenient to visit each room in turn, and have the patient demonstrate the activities usually carried out there, moving through the home by degrees. To be carried out thoroughly, the time taken will be proportionate to the gravity and number of difficulties to be overcome. Although time-consuming, such visits should be seen as part of the patient's total rehabilitation, and not as an interruption to the schedule.

The written report of the visit should be prepared as soon as possible after the event, while recall remains vivid, and so that copies can be circulated to all relevant parties in good time for their responsibilities to be actioned. There should be congruity in the measurements reported, and all converted to metric units rather than imperial wherever possible. Only the team members who have actually seen the dwelling will have an accurate first-hand picture of difficulties facing the patient at home, yet much circumstantial detail will be irrelevant to remedying them. To present a full account of the layout of the home, sketch-maps are useful visual aids, but these are seldom found in the final report. Where structural alterations are to be made, the drawing up of detailed accurate diagrams may have to be undertaken by someone other than the original assessors, depending on the disciplines represented on the visit. A scale plan is the preferred method.

An introduction to the report will give the usual file details:

— name of patient
— identification number
— address
— date of birth

This will be followed by particulars of the visit:

- date
- members of hospital staff listed by name and profession
- members of community staff similarly listed
- names of others present, and in what capacity
- main purpose of the visit
- brief note of housing type, terms of tenancy, etc.

The report should include all the requirements arising from the findings, with an indication of the referral destination, so that each staff member reading the report will know what action they in particular should take. Tactful wording of recommendations will ensure that no-one is given directives by other (perhaps junior) members of other disciplines, but that the reports are seen as problem lists and referral tools from one specific point of view to other expertise and resources. It is useful for the findings to be tabulated in columns under the headings: *Problems, Action, Referral.* A short summary and an indication of the predicted success of discharge, given the intervention listed, completes the report which should be signed by the person(s) who wrote it. A top copy should be filed in the patient's case-notes and copies sent to the individuals concerned, which may include the GP, the community nurse, the family, and perhaps the patient, according to the case in question.

SUMMARY

This chapter describes the work of the multidisciplinary team, and the particular contribution of some of its members, in organising and carrying out a combined assessment of the home and the patient, to achieve successful rehabilitation by anticipating and solving problems. The indications for such a visit, the planning and procedures are outlined step-by-step, with discussion of some of the issues and possible results, to present a comprehensive practical working guide to the subject, with suggested further reading as referenced in the text.

REFERENCES

Barber, J.H. (1984) Screening and surveillance of the elderly at risk. *The Practitioner, 228,* 269

Barker, J. and Bury, M. (1978) Mobility and the elderly: a community challenge. In V. Carver and P. Liddiard (eds), *An Ageing Population*. Open University Press with Hodder and Stoughton, Sevenoaks, 179–92

Chambers, P. (1986) Paid neighbours improve care for frail elderly. *Geriatric Medicine, 16*, 11, 42–5

Fox, D. (1981) Housing and the elderly. In D. Hobman (ed.), *The Impact of Ageing*. Croom Helm, London, 86–108

Griffiths, T. (1973) *Enjoy Your Retirement*. David and Charles, Newton Abbott

Haworth, R.J. and Hollings, E.M. (1979) Are hospital assessments of daily living activites valid? *International Journal of Rehabilitative Medicine, 1*, 59–62

Herbst, K.J. and Humphrey, C. (1980) Hearing impairment and mental state in the elderly living at home. *British Medical Journal, 281*, 903

Hill-Tout, M.L. (undated) *A Guide for Setting Up a CB Network for the Elderly in Town or Country*. From the author, The Vicarage, Horsted Keynes, Sussex

Howell, T.H. (1986) Every GP must come to terms with the 'dragons' of old age. *Geriatric Medicine, 16*, 8

Jarnlo, G.B., Ceder, L. and Thorngren, K.G. (1984) Early rehabilitation at home of elderly patients with hip fractures and consumption of resources in primary care. *Scandinavian Journal of Primary Health Care, 2*, 105

Jordan, D. (1978) Poverty and the elderly. In V. Carver and V. Liddiard, (eds), *An Ageing Population*. Open University Press with Hodder and Stoughton, Sevenoaks, 166–78

Kramer, A.M., Shaughnessy, P.W. and Pettigrew, M.L. (1985) Cost-effectiveness implications based on a comparison of nursing home and home health case mix. *Health Service Research, 20*, 387

Kübler-Ross, E. (1970) *On Death and Dying*. Tavistock, London

Lundgren-Lindquist, B., Grimby, G. and Landahl, S. (1983) Functional studies in 79-year-olds, 1. Performance in hygiene activities. *Scandinavian Journal of Rehabilitation, 15*, 109

Macmillan, D. (1960) *Lancet*, 2, 1439

Mahoney, F.I. and Barthel, D.W. (1965) Functional evaluation: the Barthel Index. *Maryland State Medical Journal, 14*, 61–5

Marshall, J. (1987) Narrated by Meades, J. in *The Victorian House*, ITV Channel 4, 28 May

Rosenblatt, D.E., Campion, E.W. and Mason, M. (1986) Rehabilitation Home Visits. *Journal of the American Geriatric Society, 34*, 441

Rossman, I. (1983) Comprehensive functional assessment: A commentary. *Journal of the American Geriatric Society, 31*, 763

Rubenstein, L.Z., Schairer, C., Wieland, G.D. and Kane, R. (1984) Systematic biases in functional status assessment of elderly adults: effects of different data sources. *Journal of Gerontology, 39*, 686

Sanford, J.R.A. (1975) Tolerance of debility in elderly dependents by supporters at home: its significance for hospital practice. *British Medical Journal, 3*, 471

Sheikh, K., Smith, D.S., Meade, T., Goldenberg, F., Brennau, P.J. and Kinsella, G. (1979) Repeatability and validity of a modified ADL index in studies of chronic disability. *International Journal of Rehabilitative Medicine, 1* 51–58

Squires, A. (1984) Checklist for a smoother and safe car trip. *Therapy Weekly*, 11, 20

Swinburne, A.C. (1865) Atalanta in Calydon. In D.K. Roberts (comp.) *The Century's Poetry 1837–1937, Vol. 1*. Penguin Books, Harmondsworth, (1938), 155–7

Trombly, A.C. and Scott, A.D. (1977) Home evaluation. In *Occupational Therapy for Physical Dysfunction*. Williams and Wilkins, Baltimore and London, 399–406

Turner, A. (1981) Home visits. In *The Practice of Occupational Therapy*. Churchill Livingstone, Edinburgh, 116–24

12

Community Physiotherapy for Elderly Patients

Thelma Harvey and Marion Judd

This chapter deals with the specific problems of elderly people living at home which require physiotherapy advice or treatment. The elderly person living in the community either at home or in an institution is often beset with multiple pathology. In addition there can be problems related to unsuitable housing, lack of heating, inadequate uptake of welfare benefits, isolation and depression which contribute to poor functional levels and increased risk of ill-health and accidents. It is proposed to discuss here those specific problems which come within the remit of the community physiotherapist.

Community physiotherapy is a relatively new branch of the profession. Community physiotherapy services gradually developed, starting in the early 1970s in response to changes and developments within the profession and the identification of the needs of patients for different and more effective methods of rehabilitation.

The enlarging of focus from hospital to include the community has highlighted the need for a realistic approach towards the patient in his own home. This means the interdependency of medical, social and psychological factors in rehabilitation to achieve the optimum level of patient function. The community physiotherapist has had to look outside her basic training to acquire new skills in understanding the personal and social needs of her patients. Working in the community, she has learned to employ a deeper level of inter-disciplinary collaboration and co-operation.

Community physiotherapy services are spread throughout the United Kingdom, but differ widely in their remit. Community physiotherapists are employed by their district health authority in the main, although a few are attached to GP practices. Some community physiotherapy services are advisory only, others offer advice and treatment. Some services are generic, some are for adults only whilst others are specifically for the elderly. Referrals countrywide come mainly from GPs. Other common sources of referral are hospital consultants, hospital physiotherapists, occupational therapists and district nurses. A community physiotherapy service may limit its referrals by accepting referrals from GPs only, or it may operate an open referral system.

STROKES

Some elderly stroke victims may be cared for entirely at home and the community physiotherapist's job is to help the patient towards optimum function. She will also spend a great deal of time advising and teaching the carers the best way to position and handle the patient. She will liaise with the GP, with the district nurse, the social worker (who may initiate a home help) and Meals-on-Wheels and the local authority occupational therapist (OT) for the provision of any aids necessary.

If the home circumstances are not adequate for the patient to be rehabilitated at home the community physiotherapist may refer the patient to hospital for physiotherapy treatment. Later it may be possible to refer the patient on to a local stroke club. Referrals may also be received for patients with previous strokes whose mobility may be deteriorating or for other specific problems. Using a problem-solving approach the community physiotherapist will identify and address the problems. This could involve a further course of treatment, a referral to a day centre or stroke club, a change of footwear, the provision of a walking aid or referral to the OT for rehousing or the social worker for rehousing in sheltered accommodation.

FRACTURES/INJURIES

The elderly person newly discharged from hospital following treatment for a fracture can be referred straight on to the community physiotherapist for continuing rehabilitation. Walking aids are reviewed, treatment, advice and teaching can be offered. Rehabilitation is geared specifically to the patient's lifestyle and environment, with progressive goal-setting until optimum function is achieved.

CHEST CONDITIONS

The community physiotherapist deals with both acute and chronic chest conditions. The most common conditions seen in United Kingdom inner city areas are chronic obstructive airways disease with acute or chronic chest infection, asthma, bronchiectasis and carcinoma of the lung. Patients tend to divide into two groups; those that need occasional treatment (e.g. during an acute episode of chest infection) and those that need regular treatment or monitoring (e.g. if they are using home nebulisers or an oxygen concentrator or use many cylinders of home oxygen a week).

With all these chest patients the main aim is to prevent the need for hospital admission by helping the patient to clear secretions and ensure the correct use of nebulisers, rotahalers, puffers, oxygen, etc.

AMPUTEES

The newly discharged elderly amputee can be seen by the physiotherapist at home. The aims of treatment will be to continue the rehabilitation started in the hospital and to monitor the patient's progress. Transfer techniques can be related to the home situation, lifting and handling can be taught to the carers if necessary. Any need for adaptations can be referred to the local authority OTs and there may be liaison with the local limb-fitting centre to ensure that the limb is fitted, and is functioning correctly. It may be necessary to refer back to the hospital out-patient department or the day hospital for further rehabilitation if this is best accomplished outside the home environment. On a long-term basis the patient may need to be seen at intervals at home to deal with any changes in mobility and function.

EARLY DISCHARGE

The elderly patient who either discharges himself or is discharged early following an illness or injury can continue his rehabilitation at home provided there is an adequate community physiotherapy service in the district. Community physiotherapy should not be used as an excuse to discharge patients too early.

LONG-TERM CHRONIC SICK

For those patients suffering from CVA, multiple sclerosis, Parkinsons's disease and other long-term or progressive neurological illnesses the community physiotherapist can:

— assess at intervals and treat or advise on specific problems
— offer regular top-up treatment
— teach carers handling techniques
— liaise with other disciplines in order to deal with problems outside her remit
— put the patient in touch with self-help groups or the relevant association for their particular disease which can give the patient additional information, help and support

Ideally, the community physiotherapist should be involved in self-help groups to teach maintenance exercises and self-care.

OSTEOARTHRITIS/RHEUMATOID ARTHRITIS

Many elderly people living at home suffer from the effects of these diseases. The community physiotherapist can initiate a programme of exercises and joint care in order to maintain mobility. These patients may need to be monitored for many years. Top-up treatment for pain relief and reassessment will be needed at intervals. Advice on walking aids and mobility generally is given. It is often necessary to assess for the correct type of wheelchair. Referral on to the local authority OTs for aids and adaptations is very common in this group of patients.

FALLS

Reasons for falling are many and complex. Taken at a very basic level, if the problem can be identified the treatment should be geared to solving that problem. Exercises to strengthen muscles and strategies for avoiding falls may be taught. Walking aids may be provided. The patient will be taught how to get up from the floor. Hazards in the home which could cause falls can be removed with the patient's agreement. Often loose mats are the culprit and can be

taken up and put away. However, on subsequent visits the physiotherapist may well find them all returned to their previous places!

GUIDELINES ON COMMUNITY PHYSIOTHERAPY FOR ELDERLY PEOPLE

In order to operate an effective community physiotherapy service for
elderly people there are specific guidelines of good practice which
should be followed:

(i) The patient must be assessed and the assessment adequately
recorded. This initial assessment will then enable the physiotherapist to identify which problems require physiotherapy
intervention or advice and a treatment programme can be
planned with the patient's agreement. Goal-setting is helpful
in reaching the final aim of treatment.

(ii) The ability to listen effectively to the patient enables the
physiotherapist to accurately identify what needs to be done
and also to be sure that this is in line with the patients' needs
and wishes.

(iii) The physiotherapist's awareness of non-physiotherapy
problems will enable her to refer the patient on to the appropriate agencies. This is very important to ensure the holistic
care of the patient whose problems are often multiple. It is
the responsibility of the community physiotherapist to be
aware of services and facilities in her health district.

(iv) Attention must be paid to the needs of the carers and
appropriate lifting and handling techniques taught, helping to
avoid back and joint problems.

(v) The community physiotherapist must inform the patients and
carers exactly how much and what type of treatment and/or
advice she is able to provide. For example, it should be
made clear that either treatment will be for a short period
until the current problem is resolved or that it will be long-
term and monitored at regular stated intervals.

(vi) The community physiotherapist must reserve the right to
refuse to provide further treatment. This is often very
difficult in the face of community pressures. The other side
of the coin is that, equally, patients have the right to refuse
to accept treatment and this must be respected.

TYPES OF ACCOMMODATION

The majority of the elderly population are housed in the same way as the general population. There are, in addition, alternative types of accommodation that are specific to the elderly. Two broad bands of types of accommodation can be identified — private and public.

Private accommodation

Elderly people living with relatives Emotional conflicts apart, these elderly are amongst the more comfortably housed providing the relatives are fit and able and well-housed themselves.

Owner-occupiers of houses These are elderly people living alone or with an equally elderly spouse. Again, if they are reasonably affluent and the house is in good repair, they can be very comfortable in this situation. It is far more usual however for the house to be in need of repair. A common picture is a leaking roof so the top floor is abandoned; a basement with very steep steps which cannot be managed; lack of adequate damp course so there is rising damp and very often dry rot is present as well. Many of these old people have managed through the years with inadequate heating, often still having coal fires, poor kitchen facilities, cold or non-existent bathrooms and outside toilets. These are all factors which cause enormous problems for elderly people. They either cannot afford improvements or could not tolerate the upheaval the work would cause. There may be a risk of hypothermia if the heating is inadequate. They are vulnerable to burglary and attack. Their house, even if they wanted to, would be difficult to sub-let because of the poor state of repair and they are usually very reluctant to sell.

These kinds of conditions apply equally to urban or rural dwellers except that in rural areas there is the added problem of lack of transport, making the elderly even more isolated.

Owner-occupiers of flats These people may be better housed, as blocks of private flats tend to be jointly serviced and decorated. The problems here are being housed on a high floor, if there is no lift, and concern about people being able to get into the block un-challenged. An entry phone system can solve this latter problem.

Private rented accommodation Very often those elderly people housed in private rented accommodation have been there for years. All that has been said about owner-occupied houses is equally applicable to this kind of dwelling.

Tied cottages There are still a large number of these in existence, often in the middle of nowhere, which can be idyllic for younger people but a nightmare for the elderly. At least the local council is obliged to rehouse these tenants if they can no longer cope.

Alms houses This ancient form of sheltered housing run by charitable trusts can still be found both in rural and urban areas. The dwellings can be quaint, have a preservation order on them, and be very cold. They can also be extremely well maintained and the residents often have a strong community spirit.

Lodgings Some people spend all their lives as a lodger and then either they or their landlady become old and no longer able to cope. Sometimes they have become so much a part of the family that other family members take them over and look after them. Others are candidates for sheltered housing or Part III accommodation.

Hotels and residential guest houses Some elderly people with means successfully make their homes in this type of accommodation.

Private sheltered housing schemes There are many such schemes being built all throughout the United Kingdom. Some are a purely commercial venture whilst others are charity-based. All are dependent for success on either a resident warden or an efficient centrally controlled alarm system.

Private residential homes The Registered Homes Act, 1984, and regulations made under the Act make provision for the registration and inspection of residential care homes offering both board and personal care for four or more persons. These regulations deal with the running of the home and the provision of services but do not specify the level of staffing needed to ensure the comfort of residents.

Local authorities are empowered to make arrangements for the placement of elderly people that are their responsibility in these homes. This usually happens when there is not sufficient number of

Part III places supplied by the local authority. Some homes will only take fairly fit elderly people, then problems arise if they become ill or too disabled for the staff of the home to manage. These residents are then often transferred to a long-stay geriatric ward or to a private nursing home. There are a few schemes where the homes are grouped so that the fitter elderly go into the first grade needing little care. As they become more disabled they are able to receive more care and finally can go to a sick bay where they are nursed. This is an excellent idea because the resident is still in familiar surroundings and can maintain the same relationships to the end.

Private nursing homes Local authority environmental health officers generally have the power to inspect premises with regard to fire safety and food hygiene. These homes may vary widely in levels of staffing, care and comfort. If the elderly person has no financial means supplementary benefit legislation provides for financial assistance towards board and lodging charges. This will usually mean sharing a ward and having little or no privacy.

Public sector accommodation

The chief advantage for the elderly living in this type of accommodation is that it is usually easier to get rehoused, sometimes into specialised housing.

Council owned houses Should be kept in reasonable state of repair but in practice such accommodation is often cold and damp.

Council owned flats These can range from well-maintained blocks with entry phone systems and adequate lifts to tower blocks that have poor, often vandalised, lifts and no security of entry phones. Elderly tenants are often afraid to be rehoused to a more suitable ground-floor flat for fear of break-ins.

Mobility housing This is really just a very good standard of building with plenty of room in corridors, bathrooms, etc. This would be suitable for an elderly person walking with a frame and should also be adequate for wheelchair users.

Wheelchair housing This is designed specifically for a permanent wheelchair user. As this is a scarce resource it is usual practice to offer a limited tenancy. For example, if the wheelchair user predeceased the more able spouse he/she would agree to be rehoused to free the property for reallocation.

Sheltered housing Throughout the United Kingdom local authority sheltered housing provision is patchy with large variations in the level of provision. Tenants have the same rights as any other council tenants and the same rights to social service department provisions (e.g. home helps, Meals-on-Wheels).

In most authorities the wardens are employed by the housing, in others by the social services department. Warden support means that there is always someone on call if a tenant needs help. Other help wardens may give depends largely on their personal abilities and willingness.

Alarm systems and peripatetic wardens Some local authorities funding blocks of flats with large numbers of elderly tenants initiate an alarm system. Each flat is wired to a central control manned by teams of peripatetic wardens who are alerted if the elderly person needs help. These are excellent schemes since no moving is required and a sense of security is maintained.

Special sheltered housing This is a provision for the more dependent tenant within a sheltered housing scheme. There may be a whole block devoted to this provision or a few beds in an ordinary sheltered housing scheme. Care staff are available to help tenants in all activities of daily living so that even heavily-dependent residents can be maintained at home.

Local authority old people's homes Part III accommodation

Only 2 per cent of the elderly population are in residential care. Sometimes these homes are purpose-built. Sometimes they are adapted, large old houses which appear more homely but present numerous obstacles for less able residents. It is very difficult for 40 to 90 old, frail strangers to live together amicably. Some residents succeed and make new friends and even marry. In smaller rural communities it is often easier as most people know one another and the home is still in the village or small town. If an elderly person can possibly be maintained at home it is better that he stays there if that is his wish.

EQUIPMENT FOR THE ELDERLY IN THE COMMUNITY

The community physiotherapist will need to have access to a supply of equipment in order to provide appropriate walking aids for her patients. Many elderly patients referred will need only a walking stick. These can be wooden, metal or have shaped handles for problem hands. It is preferable to supply a wooden stick if possible as this will last the patient's life time. The community physiotherapist needs to carry a small hacksaw in order to cut sticks to the correct height and will also need a supply of ferrules of various sizes. Patients who lean heavily on their stick may require frequent replacement of ferrules and it is often a good idea to give these patients several at a time. A stiff ferrule can be removed by gripping it in a door and twisting the stick. Metal sticks tend to become very noisy in time and a rhythmic clanking heralds the approach of the person using one which reduces their privacy. However, for some elderly hands the grip on a metal stick is more comfortable and therefore this will be the stick of choice to prescribe.

The community physiotherapist will also need access to a large variety of walking frames in order to optimise patient function. Adjustable frames are needed to cater for different heights of patients. The width of frame is especially important for use at home. Folding frames are used for those permanent frame-users who go out regularly by car. More specialised frames may be needed such as rollators, gutter rollators and frames which have a seat as an integral part of the frame. Many patients use a small trolley successfully between kitchen and living room instead of their frame when they want to carry food or drink in from the kitchen to the table. A net bag to fasten on to the frame is also useful for the permanent frame-user to carry belongings about in. The patient who lives in a house with internal stairs may need to be issued with two frames — one for downstairs and one for upstairs — giving access to the whole of the house. Some patients may need to be issued with crutches. This can be either a temporary supply following an injury or, more usually, it is a replacement for old crutches which have worn out. Underarm crutches are very popular with some groups of users such as old polio victims and some amputees use an underarm crutch instead of an artificial limb. Sometimes they refuse to part with their original crutch and this has to be re-upholstered. The patient with osteoarthritic spine or cervical spondylosis with nerve root pressure will require a collar either ready-made or made to measure. Some patients may need night collars. There are many commercially manufactured collars on the market, or the community physiotherapist may wish to make her own where appropriate.

If elderly patients have not had their orthotic needs catered for in hospital the community physiotherapist can assess and refer the patient back to the hospital for appropriate splinting or supply and fit ready-made splinting herself. She may find it necessary to make some splints in the patient's home. Elderly people who need specialised footwear and have been referred to the community physiotherapist from hospital may have already had their footwear needs organised. This is not a very common occurrence. If the community physiotherapist takes GP referrals she will immediately come across a large section of the elderly population with multiple foot problems and difficulty in finding suitable footwear. The patient may need to be referred on to the chiropody service, as a first contact by the physiotherapist will often bring to light problems with overgrown toenails and painful corns which detract from the patient's ability to walk.

In order to function optimally elderly people may need aids for daily living. Most commonly the helping hand, long-handled shoe-horn, high armchair, bed raisers, Roma trolleys and bath aids are required. The community physiotherapist will refer the patient on to the social services occupational therapist for assessment and provision of these aids. The occupational therapist will also assess for handrails, structural alterations and rehousing if necessary. The community physiotherapist may refer to the district nursing service for nursing aids. Most commonly needed are sheepskins, bed pans, urinals, ripple mattresses and ripple cushions.

The community physiotherapist can assess for and order wheelchairs through the patient's GP and the local artificial limb and appliance centre. The provision of a wheelchair for infirm and elderly patients to enable them to be taken out can add immeasurably to their quality of life. The community physiotherapist is a resource for the elderly person with difficulty in finding suitable clothing. For complex dressing problems the physiotherapist can obtain information from the Disabled Living Foundation and pass on advice to the patient or refer the patient on to an occupational therapist.

THE ROLE OF THE COMMUNITY PHYSIOTHERAPIST IN TEACHING AND PREVENTION

The role of the community physiotherapist in teaching and prevention is threefold.

First, her job is to teach the patient how best to cope with his/her disability. This involves teaching walking skills, transferring techniques, ways of functioning within the home environment and exercise programmes to improve function. The success of physiotherapy treatment depends greatly on the ability to teach the patient effectively.

Secondly, the physiotherapist will be involved in teaching relatives and carers how to handle the patient and how to avoid back problems.

Thirdly, the community physiotherapist is a resource for other members of the multidisciplinary team and should be available to advise and teach fellow professionals.

With the growing emphasis on community care and the projected rise in the elderly population more and more health education and prevention information is being provided for the public and is increasingly being planned as part of a package for community care. There are several prime areas where the community physiotherapist can make a contribution. The traditional role of physiotherapy in preventative work has been in back care and teaching lifting and handling techniques and this role continues with patients, carers and fellow professionals. In addition, community physiotherapists are increasingly taking part in pre-retirement groups where they teach a variety of preventative techniques. These include keep-fit exercises, care of joints and prevention of deformity, care of feet and advice on how to keep them functional, advice on footwear, advice on chest care, incontinence and help with stopping smoking. Involvement with younger anti-smoking groups will help to prevent smoking-related disease in old age.

Pensioners' groups often have a health education input and, again, the community physiotherapist is a resource to advise on and teach the prevention of physical deterioration where possible. In addition to teaching the fit elderly the community physiotherapist can give valuable input to groups of elderly disabled such as stroke clubs, day centres, etc. Her aims here will be, again, to promote optimum function and prevent further deterioration. The physiotherapist can advise clients where to seek keep fit classes run by local authorities or organisations such as Extend who exist specifically for the elderly or disabled population. Swimming classes for the elderly are held at some baths and the physiotherapist involved in preventative work will have a knowledge of local facilities which she can then pass on to her clients.

RELATIONSHIPS WITH OTHER AGENCIES IN THE COMMUNITY

The community physiotherapist has to form good relationships with those people and agencies that are most important to her patient. Table 12.1 is not meant to be exhaustive but does give some indication of the diversity of relationships that are possible.

THE COMMUNITY PHYSIOTHERAPIST AND THE LAW

As an employee of the NHS, the community physiotherapist in the United Kingdom is subject to the same legal framework as a hospital physiotherapist.

However, there are additional factors impinging on her working situation by virtue of the fact of not working within the protected environment of hospital premises, and these factors will be briefly discussed here.

Safety

Whereas it is the responsibility of the employing authority to provide a safe working environment for its employees, the community physiotherapist's work falls largely outside this environment and, therefore, the employing authority has a duty to provide training for community staff in coping with potential risks and hazards in a community setting.

Such hazards can be many and varied including faulty wiring, loose mats, collapsing stairs or furniture, violent dogs, cats, low-flying budgerigars, disturbed or violent patients, theft of physiotherapist's car or equipment, fleas, lice, being trapped in lifts, mugging, rape, etc.

A community hazard register should be maintained so that

Table 12.1: Diversity of possible relationships

Agencies frequently contacted	Agencies sometimes contacted	Agencies occasionally contacted
General practitioner	Church	Age Concern
Social worker	Welfare rights officer	Transport
Occupational therapist	Continence advisor	Community speech therapist
Home nurse	Dentist	Orthotist
Health visitor	Optician	Tenants association
Home help	Hairdresser	Dial-a-ride
Bathing attendant	District general hospital staff	ALAC limbs and wheelchairs
Volunteers	Geriatric day hospital	Vet
Chiropodists	Stroke club	Stoma advisor
Neighbours	Part III accommodation	Police
Lunch club	Special sheltered housing	Hearing aid clinic
Day centre	Terminal care team	Societies/Associations*
	Estate managers	

* Some examples will include: Multiple Sclerosis Society, Royal National Institute for the Blind, Parkinson's Disease Society, Chest, Heart and Stroke Association, Alzheimer's Disease Society

management can review hazards to which staff are exposed and can provide appropriate training. There should be a health and safety at work policy relating to the community which should be reviewed every two years. There must be a procedure for recording acccidents (e.g. an accident form to make sure that any injury is recorded at the time). Claims for criminal injury are made through the criminal injury compensation board. The police must be informed at the time of the injury.

Consent to treatment

The physiotherapist visiting an elderly patient at home may not touch the patient without his/her consent. This consent is rarely formally sought but is usually inferred from the patient's behaviour. There are three factors which constitute valid consent to treatment:

(i) Mental competence of the patient to make a decision.
(ii) Information given and received about the proposed treatment.
(iii) Voluntary agreement by the patient to accept the proposed treatment.

It is clear that an elderly person who is mentally competent has the right to refuse treatment and the community physiotherapist must respect this right.

Provision of services

The community physiotherapist has a duty to formally raise the issue of excessive case load with her manager. The manager has a duty to stop the service rather than provide an inadequate service — which can open the way to claims of negligence. Referrals should not be accepted if no treatment is available because of staff shortages; otherwise the client could sue the health authority. If the referral cannot be accepted the referrer should be told.

Records

Records are legal documents and need to be an accurate statement of fact, not judgemental or humorous.

Gifts

Gifts are legally the property of the employing authority. Gifts should not be accepted. If accepted they should be recorded. There should be a policy on gifts from the employing authority.

Conclusion

It is in the interest of the community physiotherapist to obtain full information on her legal status from her employing authority before commencing her job.

SUMMARY

Community physiotherapy for elderly patients embraces a whole range of skills and roles. In line with current trends towards community care for elderly people, and as a member of the multidisciplinary team in the community, the physiotherapist has a valuable contribution to make towards the care of the elderly at home.

13

Community Occupational Therapy for Elderly People

Jean Hall

This chapter is written from the viewpoint of a practising occupational therapist, with experience of working in a range of hospital settings and in an Outer London borough's social services department.

The role of the occupational therapist in such a setting has developed considerably since 1970 with the enactment of the Chronically Sick and Disabled Persons Act 1970, and has been accelerated by the passage of the Disabled Persons (Services, Consultation and Representation) Act 1986. (See Appendix I.)

Working in social services provides a rich assortment of experience, ranging from very basic services, such as providing advice to clients and/or their carer(s) on practical ways of adapting to altered circumstances resulting from illness, disability or general frailty, to that of providing a full rehabilitation/resettlement programme which will enable disabled persons to live independently in the community and, wherever possible, in their own home.

The role of the occupational therapist working in a social services department of a local authority is different from, but complementary to, that of his/her colleague working in a hospital. Whilst the hospital-based occupational therapist will be responsible for treatment and rehabilitation programmes, the social services occupational therapist will be responsible for resettlement if the patient is being discharged home, and for facilitating independent living or care with dignity for that patient/client.

The terminology is worth noting here: the hospital 'patient' becomes social services 'client' once discharge has been established. It is worth noting, too, that only a relatively small proportion of referrals are directly from hospital. The majority of clients are referred by GPs, district nurses, relatives, neighbours, home helps, or may request assistance for themselves. All referrals will be considered, but only accepted on the assurance that the person being referred concurs with this.

The responsibilities of the occupational therapist working for a local authority social services department will vary in both range and quality from one local authority to another within the United Kingdom.

These differences will depend upon such things as:

- the size of the local authority
- whether it is a borough or a county council
- the political colour of the local authority
- the commitment of the elected members on the social services committee and of the officers to meeting the needs of disabled persons and to the employment of occupational therapists
- availability of suitably qualified occupational therapists, given the national shortfall of qualified staff

The common link between occupational therapists, whether hospital- or social services-based, and between colleagues in the other paramedical professions, is the dedication to the welfare and independence of their clients or patients. Before going into specific details of cases and examples of working practice, it is advisable to explain that there are no national standardised procedures for the provision of services to disabled persons. Occupational therapists make every attempt to keep abreast of new ideas, techniques, policies and practice by means of discussion, exchange of papers and training sessions. There are a number of forums where examples of practice, good and not so good, are discussed and illustrated, and where highly motivated professionals and people with disabilities are able to influence standards and practice at all levels. These include special interest groups, the London Boroughs' Occupational Therapist Managers' Group, Centre on Environment for the Handicapped, The Disabled Living Foundation and independent living centres around the United Kingdom. Politicians and members of public bodies are invaluable in providing a two-way exchange of information which can influence the legislators and policy makers.

Because there are no nationally agreed standards of service provision in the United Kingdom, there are large differences between local authorities in range and quality of services for disabled persons. The examples of service provision given below are therefore not necessarily representative of all local authorities. Reference will be made, as appropriate, to the changes which are expected as the Disabled Persons' (Services, Consultation and Representation) Act 1986 is implemented.

THE ROLE OF THE LOCAL AUTHORITY OCCUPATIONAL THERAPIST

This covers a number of aspects:

(i) To assist in providing a service to clients, who may be disabled, elderly or recovering from illness, enabling them to live as independently as possible and, where appropriate, with care and dignity.

(ii) To act as a departmental professional adviser on matters relating to disability, liaising where necessary with individuals or groups of disabled people.

(iii) To take referrals and to deal with them appropriately; this may be in providing advice to disabled clients and/or their families. It may mean long-term involvement in casework and in coordinating services which will facilitate independent living.

(iv) To visit disabled persons, to carry out assessments of their abilities, short-term and long-term needs, and to make recommendations accordingly.

(v) To make careful note of the abilities and difficulties which the carer(s) may be having. This will take on greater importance with the implementation of Section 8(1) of the Disabled Persons' Act 1986.

(vi) To carefully record and report at all stages. This is necessary in order to check progress and to ensure that proposed action is taken. Such supervision ensures that facts can be ascertained in the event of a query or dispute. In the event of staff changes, clear records facilitate a smooth changeover and reduce 'hassle' for client and therapist. Where, as in the installation of major house adaptations, considerable financial implications may be involved, it is essential that details are accurately recorded and dated for a possible audit inspection.

(vii) To set in motion and follow through such action as has been agreed by the client and, where necessary, by senior members of staff in a supervisory capacity.

(viii) To record those needs which have been identified but which cannot immediately be met by existing services, and to draw this information to the attention of managers or members of other council departments, if it is considered that services for other clients may be improved.

An example of this could be to identify the need for more sheltered housing for older clients. By keeping accurate records of those elderly persons who wish to move into accommodation, which provides the security of 24-hour surveillance by a resident warden, and by transmitting this information to the housing department, plans can be prepared for rehousing those people.

Where there is an identified shortfall between need and availability of suitable housing, the director of housing can take action. This may take the form of reporting to committee and obtaining the necessary funding for building more units, or it may involve negotiations with housing associations to build more units for sale or rent.

The more enlightened management or major projects staff in housing departments involve the occupational therapists and representatives from local disability groups in the planning, location and design of 'special' housing. It is also good practice to consult the occupational therapist when considering the suitability of a particular unit of accommodation for a disabled, elderly client. Sometimes, where clients are desperate to move, they will accept something which they see as a vast improvement on their existing accommodation, and will be oblivious to the potential difficulties with which they will be faced if it is impracticable for their use. A small number of local authority social service departments have appointed occupational therapists to work with the staff in the housing department to deal specifically with 'special needs' housing.

REFERRALS

A referral may be made by anyone; the client, a relative, neighbour or friend, the coalman or milkman, anyone in fact who is concerned for the welfare of another person. A referral will be accepted only where the person being referred knows that a referral is being made and is agreeable. In most cases a referral will only be accepted where adequate supporting information can be given.

The occupational therapist should have access to the client's GP and should keep him/her informed of progress, or otherwise. All information relating to the clients must be treated as confidential. In complex cases or where it is necessary to seek guidance on the likely prognosis of a patient/client it may be necessary for the occupational therapist to seek more detailed advice from the client's medical consultant.

Occasionally, conflicting viewpoints between medical advisers and/or the client and social services will cause difficulties. In these cases it may be necessary for the OT to ask the community medical officer, who has responsibility for liaison between the health authority and the local authority, to mediate.

Careful documentation of all referrals is essential and local administrative requirements will dictate the layout of referral forms and the details required. Many local authorities are putting such information on computers, which facilitates access by more than one agency. The need for absolute confidentiality must be emphasised. This is underpinned by the legislation of the 1984 Data Protection Act. This requires the users, as individuals who are responsible for the input of information, to keep that information updated, and to be responsible for the confidential safekeeping of such information including printouts.

It is essential that the details recorded on a referral are absolutely accurate and as informative as possible. Good office procedure should ensure that anyone receiving a referral appreciates the principles involved, and understands the importance of accurate listening, questioning and recording.

WAITING LISTS AND PRIORITIES

Referrals are recorded by date and given priority according to urgency indicated by information provided. Allocation systems vary according to location, staffing levels and local policies. Where there are a number of occupational therapists it is preferable to have a senior who has responsibility for allocation and supervision. In busy departments where referrals are received at a faster rate than they can be actioned, this method relieves the occupational therapist of some of the anxiety and pressure. It is advisable for ongoing records to be kept of all referrals, numbers and type, for statistical support when making bids for additional staff and for improvements or changes in resource allocation. Optimum case loads will vary according to experience and workstyle of the occupational therapist, and on the complexity of the individual case work.

Practice regarding the 'opening' and 'closure' of cases will vary. Some occupational therapists prefer to close a case once they have completed a piece of work with a client. Other therapists will keep a case open where there is likely to be ongoing, but intermittent involvement. There are no hard and fast rules but a case load for a reasonably mature and experienced occupational therapist is likely to average 50 of varying complexity.

ASSESSMENT

The importance of the assessment cannot be over-emphasised. The way in which this is carried out from the referral stage is important not only for its accuracy and attention to detail, but also for the way in which it is transacted.

The majority of clients will be visited at home. However, some will be visited before being discharged from hospital or from a residential establishment such as a special school, hostel or specialist unit. The first visit should be arranged by telephone, if possible, and followed by a confirmatory letter, signed clearly by the occupational therapist, explaining the purpose of the visit, the time and likely duration.

The planned visit should go as arranged and to time. If a delay is unavoidable, every attempt should be made to notify the client in reasonable time and to allow for their plans. The therapist should be considerate in the way s/he makes the first visit, and should be sensitive to the lifestyle and wishes of the client. The listening and observation skills of the therapist are as important as the way in which rapport is established between therapist and client and, where appropriate, clients' family, neighbour or home help.

Methods of recording an assessment will vary according to different workstyles. Some people prefer to work to a standard format or *aide mémoire*. Others prefer to work to a programme which they memorise. Whichever method is used, it is very important now, and will be of even greater importance as the implications of Sections 3 and 4 of the Disabled Persons Act 1986 are realised, to ensure accuracy of factual material and to ensure that observations and conclusions are well and logically supported.

These implications are clearly spelt out in a Royal Association of Disability and Rehabilitation (RADAR) document (July 1986):

Section 3: Assessment by local authorities of the needs of disabled persons.

This section requires local authorities, before making an assessment of the need of a disabled person for any social services provision, to allow him or his authorised representative to make representations as to his needs. At the request of the disabled person or his authorised representative the authority must provide a written statement of their decision specifying:

the needs accepted by the authority and the services they propose to provide to meet them; or

that in their opinion the disabled person has no needs; and

the reasons for their decision.

If they (the local authority) do not propose to provide a service to meet a need identified by the disabled person or his authorised representative, they must also state this and explain the reasons.

A right of the disabled person or his authorised representative to ask for a review of any decision is included in the section. Assistance must be given during the assessment procedures if either the disabled person or his authorised representative is unable to communicate on account of disability.

Section 4: Services under Section 2 of the 1970 Act: duty to consider the needs of disabled persons.

This section confirms that a local authority must assess the need of a disabled person for any of the services listed in Section 2 of the Chronically Sick and Disabled Persons Act 1970 if asked by the disabled person, his authorised representative or a carer (as defined in Section 8).

The individual viewpoints and comments of patients should be noted separately and the implications of the legislation on 'client access to information' borne in mind.

As a result of the Disabled Persons Act 1986 the format and content of assessment forms are under review. The occupational therapist must be prepared to carry out very specific and detailed assessments at the request of the client who wishes to make a formal or legal representation. Groups of local authority occupational therapists are currently preparing guidelines to ensure that therapists have all the necessary knowledge and skills to carry out such very specific assessments and that they understand the legal implications.

ASSESSMENT FOR WHAT?

Even the most carefully completed referral form will not necessarily prepare the therapist for what s/he will find on visiting. Because there are as many likely situations as there are clients, it is only possible to set down some general principles and a few examples.

The most frequent request is for assistance with bathing. This may be translated as the client having practical difficulties due to physical impairment. Assuming that the client has a bath, the difficulties may be:

— the bath is too high, too low, or slippery
— there is a need for strategically placed grabrails, bath seat, or non-slip mat
— a method of lifting the client into and out of the bath is required
— a different kind of bath, or a shower, is required
— a downstairs bath/shower room is required as the client can no longer climb stairs

On visiting, the therapist will frequently find that the client is having difficulties with activities other than bathing, but assistance has been sought with this particular activity in the interests of hygiene and safety. Clues to the client's problems may lie in the way s/he moves, time taken getting to the door and opening it, the way in which s/he sits or stands, and the condition of the house.

First impressions are important, but should be weighed carefully when interviewing the client. Assumptions should be held in check and should be voiced with care. It is all too easy to make an unguarded comment which can hinder the progress of an accurate assessment.

If, after some preliminary questioning, it is apparent that the client is having difficulties in several areas of daily activity, the therapist may proceed to make a more detailed assessment or make arrangements to call again at a more mutually convenient time. It may also be deemed necessary to consult with the client's GP, or a relative of the client, who should be present during the assessment. The degree to which a client will trust the therapist will depend very much on individual personalities and temperaments, but ultimately it is the skill of the therapist which will elicit the necessary information to make a comprehensive assessment.

WHAT ACTION IS TO FOLLOW THE ASSESSMENT?

The client's difficulty may be resolved by the therapist demonstrating and teaching a new technique in the way a particular action is carried out, or it may be that by rearranging some household furniture, with the client's agreement, the client can move more freely. Where the solution lies in providing an aid or piece of equipment which will enable the client to achieve independence, the therapist will either deliver the aid or piece of equipment and instruct the client in its safe use, or arrange for these to be carried out.

Suitable aids will not necessarily be available from stock, in which case the OT will have to investigate the source of supply of appropriate solutions. (The Information Service of the Disabled Living Foundation is an invaluable source of such information on different types of equipment, addresses of manufacturers and suppliers, prices and other useful information. This service may be obtained by annual subscription.)

It is necessary for occupational therapists to update their knowledge of available equipment and to seek detailed demonstrations where they may check for themselves the purpose and suitability of individual items. (The NAIDEX exhibitions and the Disabled Living Foundation and independent living centres are extremely valuable in this respect.)

Local policies vary over what can be provided as aids which are essential and those which are thought desirable but not essential. Charging policies also vary. Many local authorities will loan aids and equipment free of charge, only recouping the cost if the client moves to another local authority. Some local authorities make charges for certain specified items within a particular range, by price or by type of aid.

Increasingly, certain shops are keeping a stock of the more commonly requested items, and clients are encouraged to purchase from them with advice from a suitably experienced OT. Items which are commonly classified as 'sick room equipment' are usually provided by the NHS, often using the Red Cross to administer the service. More forward-looking authorities are experimenting in the setting up of joint aids/equipment stores which enable paramedical staff, whether employed by the health authority or local authority, to select and issue equipment.

It is vitally important that strict criteria and careful guidelines are agreed as to who is authorised to issue aids, and that personnel are trained and updated in all aspects of selection, safety and hygiene. As new equipment becomes available it becomes increasingly necessary to ensure standards of good, appropriate design and quality control. It is also important that administrative procedures are followed and careful records kept of issues. This is particularly important where equipment needs to be recalled or replaced, particularly if a piece of equipment has been found to be defective and dangerous. Sometimes an item is so dangerous that it is necessary to recall a complete batch of similar items.

When an aid or piece of equipment has been issued it is important that instructions are given, and understood, on its use and care, including any counter-instructions which may be necessary. It is important, too, at this stage to observe how the client uses the equipment and to ensure that its use and possible misuse is fully understood. A specific example would be a mechanical or electric hoist and slings. In this situation it is important that all members of the household understand the principles of its use and what to do in an emergency. (A memorable experience was the safe and unblushing release of a naked lady from an electrically-operated bath hoist which had stuck in the midway position. Fortunately, the lady's husband was in the house and telephoned the occupational therapist who, in turn, telephoned the Fire Brigade and then made a speedy dash, equipped with a large blanket, to meet the firemen at the client's house. After reassuring the client and her husband, the occupational therapist briefed the firemen as to what was required of them, wrapped a towel and the blanket around the lady, and she was released unharmed and unembarrassed. Once the client was comfortably settled in her wheelchair, the electrical engineer was called in to remedy the fault in the hoist mechanism. Although the hoist had been regularly and properly serviced a component had failed.)

Wherever a client is dependent upon a piece of mechanical and/or electrical equipment it is essential to have available a means of calling for assistance. Clients are advised to ensure that they have household insurance cover on equipment such as lifts, hoists and stairlifts.

ADAPTATIONS TAKE A LITTLE LONGER!

Where disabled people can no longer function independently, if at all, without making alterations to the building in which they reside, more complex solutions may be necessary. Adaptations include structural alterations which affect the fabric of the building. The ownership of the property is important, as it is necessary to obtain permission from the owner before any alterations are made. It is advisable to obtain agreement in principle before proceeding to obtain expensive plans for major adaptations.

Simple adaptations include such items as grabrails and stair rails, small ramps, alterations to individual steps, alterations to window catches, lowering or raising of shelves, installation of raised electric sockets. Major adaptations include additional downstairs facilities, such as toilets, shower/bathrooms or bedroom extensions. These are deemed necessary where the client is no longer able to go upstairs and does not wish, or cannot afford to move house. In these circumstances consideration may be given to the installation of a personal lift or a stair-lift.

The options must be considered carefully in the light of the client's physical and mental condition, lifestyle, family as well as individual needs and the wishes of all concerned. In some local authorities where budgets are slim and policies unimaginative, there is the danger that the client's best long-term interests will go unheeded and minimal provision made. This can prove to be a short-sighted and expensive process if, for example, a stairlift is installed and the client's known condition deteriorates. If this means that the stairlift has to be removed and an extension built, the long-term cost includes the installation and removal of the stairlift, plus the additional building costs of the adaptation which will be greater than if the extension had been built when the needs of the client were first identified. There is the additional hassle to the client whose condition will have deteriorated, and who will have to contend with building works and all that that entails at a time when his or her condition is less robust.

The process of getting work done will depend on such factors as type and size of adaptation. For example, a grabrail will probably be fitted by a technician employed by the local authority social services department, or by a local contractor who caters for minor works. Major adaptations will be managed by an architect or building surveyor, and estimates or tenders will be sought before the building work can be commenced.

PREPARATION FOR ADAPTATIONS

The following chart (Table 13.1) gives an indication of the range of options which may face a client. It is an example extracted from a set of procedures designed to assist the occupational therapist to find a pathway through a maze of alternatives, and to ensure that each stage of the adaptation follows smoothly.

The success of any adaptation is measured by how far it accommodates the needs of the disabled and their immediate family or carer, in improving their quality of life and independence. Important factors in achieving success will include:

(i)   The skill and imagination of the occupational therapist in carrying out a thorough and detailed assessment of the needs of the client in the short- and the long-term, and translating these into a realistic set of proposals for action.

(ii) Good rapport and communication between the occupational therapist and the client and family whilst reaching agreement on what is required.

(iii) Skilled teamwork, led by the occupational therapist, by all concerned in the design, preparation and building of the adaptation. The team will probably include an architect (preferably one who has some understanding of the specific needs of the disabled or elderly person) environmental health officer (where a home improvement grant is being sought), planning officer, finance officer/adviser, the builder, and (in council property) a member of the housing department.

(iv) Sufficient funds being available to finance the recommendations at each stage.

Table 13.1: Starting procedure for all jobs

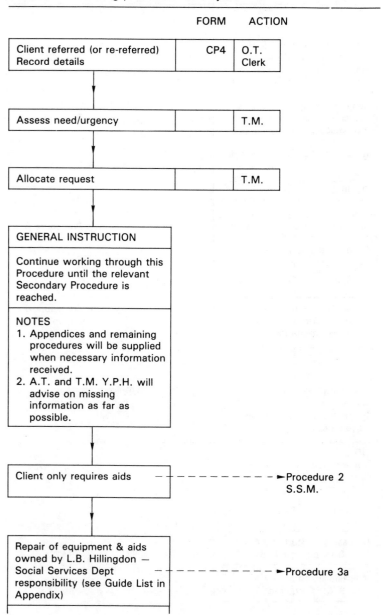

FORM   ACTION

	FORM	ACTION
Client referred (or re-referred) Record details	CP4	O.T. Clerk

Assess need/urgency		T.M.

Allocate request		T.M.

GENERAL INSTRUCTION

Continue working through this Procedure until the relevant Secondary Procedure is reached.

NOTES
1. Appendices and remaining procedures will be supplied when necessary information received.
2. A.T. and T.M. Y.P.H. will advise on missing information as far as possible.

Client only requires aids — — — — — — — — ►Procedure 2 S.S.M.

Repair of equipment & aids owned by L.B. Hillingdon — Social Services Dept responsibility (see Guide List in Appendix) — — — — — — — — ►Procedure 3a

Table 13.1 *cont.*

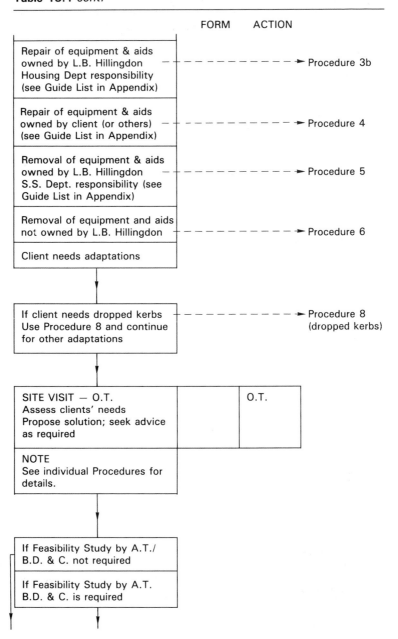

FORM   ACTION

Repair of equipment & aids owned by L.B. Hillingdon Housing Dept responsibility (see Guide List in Appendix) — — — — — — — — ➤ Procedure 3b

Repair of equipment & aids owned by client (or others) (see Guide List in Appendix) — — — — — — — — ➤ Procedure 4

Removal of equipment & aids owned by L.B. Hillingdon S.S. Dept. responsibility (see Guide List in Appendix) — — — — — — — — ➤ Procedure 5

Removal of equipment and aids not owned by L.B. Hillingdon — — — — — — — — ➤ Procedure 6

Client needs adaptations

If client needs dropped kerbs Use Procedure 8 and continue for other adaptations — — — — — — — — ➤ Procedure 8 (dropped kerbs)

SITE VISIT — O.T. Assess clients' needs Propose solution; seek advice as required | O.T.

NOTE See individual Procedures for details.

If Feasibility Study by A.T./ B.D. & C. not required

If Feasibility Study by A.T. B.D. & C. is required

Table 13.1 *cont.*

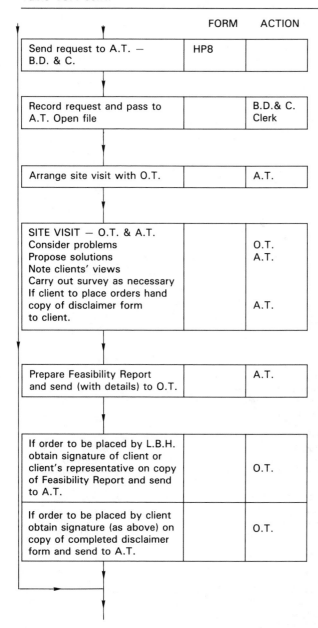

	FORM	ACTION
Send request to A.T. — B.D. & C.	HP8	
Record request and pass to A.T. Open file		B.D.& C. Clerk
Arrange site visit with O.T.		A.T.
SITE VISIT — O.T. & A.T. Consider problems Propose solutions Note clients' views Carry out survey as necessary If client to place orders hand copy of disclaimer form to client.		O.T. A.T. A.T.
Prepare Feasibility Report and send (with details) to O.T.		A.T.
If order to be placed by L.B.H. obtain signature of client or client's representative on copy of Feasibility Report and send to A.T.		O.T.
If order to be placed by client obtain signature (as above) on copy of completed disclaimer form and send to A.T.		O.T.

Table 13.1 *cont.*

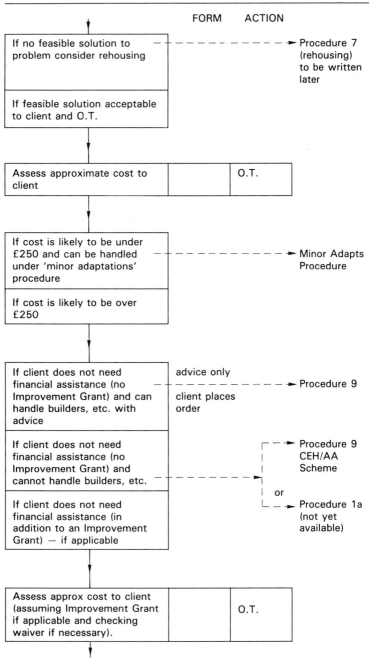

FORM   ACTION

If no feasible solution to problem consider rehousing — — — — — — — — — — ► Procedure 7 (rehousing) to be written later

If feasible solution acceptable to client and O.T.

Assess approximate cost to client   O.T.

If cost is likely to be under £250 and can be handled under 'minor adaptations' procedure — — — — — — — — — — ► Minor Adapts Procedure

If cost is likely to be over £250

If client does not need financial assistance (no Improvement Grant) and can handle builders, etc. with advice — advice only — — — — — — — — ► Procedure 9 client places order

If client does not need financial assistance (no Improvement Grant) and cannot handle builders, etc. — — — — — — — ► Procedure 9 CEH/AA Scheme or Procedure 1a (not yet available)

If client does not need financial assistance (in addition to an Improvement Grant) — if applicable

Assess approx cost to client (assuming Improvement Grant if applicable and checking waiver if necessary).   O.T.

Table 13.1 *cont.*

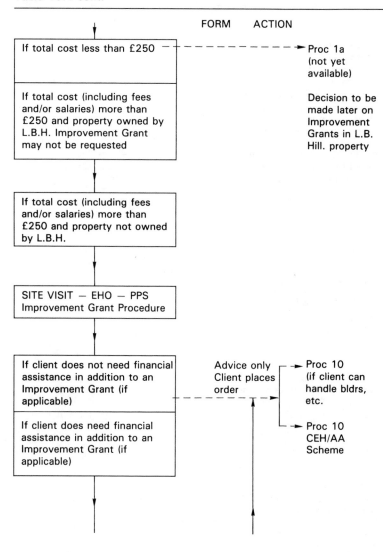

	FORM	ACTION
If total cost less than £250		Proc 1a (not yet available)
If total cost (including fees and/or salaries) more than £250 and property owned by L.B.H. Improvement Grant may not be requested		Decision to be made later on Improvement Grants in L.B. Hill. property
If total cost (including fees and/or salaries) more than £250 and property not owned by L.B.H.		
SITE VISIT — EHO — PPS Improvement Grant Procedure		
If client does not need financial assistance in addition to an Improvement Grant (if applicable)	Advice only Client places order	Proc 10 (if client can handle bldrs, etc.
If client does need financial assistance in addition to an Improvement Grant (if applicable)		Proc 10 CEH/AA Scheme

Table 13.1 *cont.*

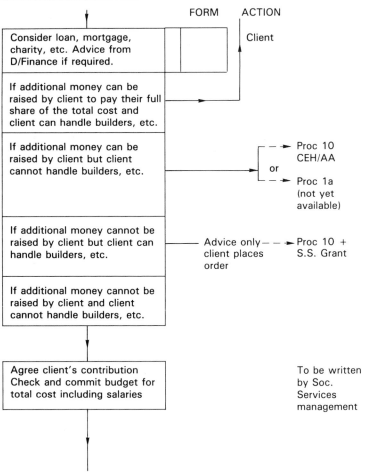

FORM   ACTION

Consider loan, mortgage, charity, etc. Advice from D/Finance if required. — Client

If additional money can be raised by client to pay their full share of the total cost and client can handle builders, etc.

If additional money can be raised by client but client cannot handle builders, etc. — Proc 10 CEH/AA or Proc 1a (not yet available)

If additional money cannot be raised by client but client can handle builders, etc. — Advice only — client places order — Proc 10 + S.S. Grant

If additional money cannot be raised by client and client cannot handle builders, etc.

Agree client's contribution Check and commit budget for total cost including salaries — To be written by Soc. Services management

Procedure 1a
(not yet available — covers Procedures not complete as decisions are still needed from Social Services Management.)

(v) Clear communications at all stages of the design and building.

(vi) Adequate preparation, both physically and psychologically, for the disruption which will inevitably occur when building works commence.

Throughout the process, the OT will be an important figure, available to give support throughout the contractual process. For example, it may be necessary to arrange respite care for the client when dust and debris or lack of water and toilet amenity will cause distress to the client and his carer. Alternatively, it may be necessary for the OT to be available to provide advice or temporary equipment, such as a chemical toilet, if the client is to remain at home while adaptations are in progress.

TEAMWORK IN GETTING ADAPTATIONS BUILT

Where it is necessary for adaptations to be made to the client's home the occupational therapist is the coordinator between numerous individual people, each a specialist in his/her own right, working as a team. This membership of the team will vary from case to case, but over a period of time, the occupational therapist will build up a valuable group of people who will be experienced in assisting clients to retain their dignity and independence.

The teamwork necessary to get a patient discharged home from hospital is outlined in Table 13.2.

Arrangements for processing adaptations will depend on local policies and practices. The Centre on Environment for the Handicapped have reports emanating from their seminars on this subject, which show that no two local authorities follow the same pattern.

Figure 13.1 shows a scale model which is used to simulate existing layouts as well as proposed plans for adaptation. The model, which was made by an architectural model maker, enables occupational therapists and their clients to discuss alternative planned layouts. This is of particular value where the available space in a building is limited and where the client is a wheelchair user.

The scale model is valuable as a teaching method, enabling students, new members of staff and clients to translate two-dimensional drawings into three-dimensional reality. It helps them to assess whether a proposed adaptation is a feasible scheme. It is also

Table 13.2: Probable teamwork necessary to get a patient home from hospital

Hospital	Working with	Social services	Other agencies
Nursing staff	Patient/client	Occupational therapist	Architect (where major adaptations are necessary)
Medical staff	Patient's family/carer	OT technician	Building surveyor (for small adaptations)
Physiotherapist	General practitioner		Planning Officer
Occupational therapist			Building control officer
Social worker			Environmental health officer (for Home Improvement Grants)
			Finance officer
			Building contractor
			Structural engineer
			Specialist installation technician
			Landlord, possibly the local Housing Department
			Legal advisor

valuable in that it sometimes prevents expensive mistakes being made (e.g. model wheelchair and bathroom hoists will highlight possible 'tight spots' on a plan) and it will also enable the client to experiment with alternative layouts and to participate in the planning process.

Figure 13.2 shows a plan of the layout of a building before and after adaptation.

THE EXTERNAL ENVIRONMENT

Occupational therapists will inevitably be involved with their clients in overcoming some of the problems of the external environment. Having ensured that a client can live independently indoors, it is logical that s/he will wish to go out, visit friends and relatives, go to shops, post office, library, pub, railway station. Where the client is dependent upon a wheelchair it is necessary to ascertain whether the pavements have sufficient dropped kerbs to enable the client to travel safely to a destination. The occupational therapist will frequently be involved in the process of getting the highways department of the relevant authority to lower kerbs at strategic crossing points. Broken paving stones, inconsistently placed street furniture, shop blinds and pavement displays of goods for sale are all contributory factors to causing accidents, particularly where a person's vision is defective.

The appalling lack of accessibility into and within public and commercial buildings continues to be a major handicap to people with mobility problems, particularly the elderly. Occupational therapists will frequently be involved in advising on improvements necessary to overcome such problems and to make recommendations on improving the design and layout of buildings. Some local authorities have introduced policies to accommodate some of the environmental needs of disabled people. An increasing number are appointing access officers, whose responsibility it is to ensure that the access requirements of the Chronically Sick and Disabled Persons Act 1970, the 1976 Amendment and the 1981 Disabled Persons Act are implemented, and that architects, builders and developers not only understand their responsibilities towards disabled persons, but do all that they can to act upon the recommendations.

There is a considerable need to improve the facilities available to assist elderly people when they are travelling, shopping or simply

Figure 13.1: Scale model used to simulate layouts. (a) and (b) illustrate the situation before adaptation, while (c) demonstrates an alternative layout

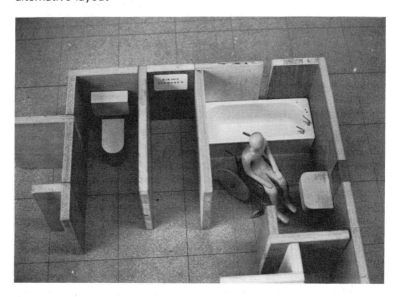

(a)

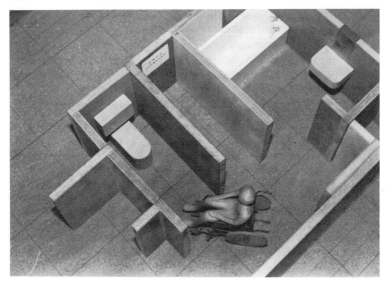

(b)

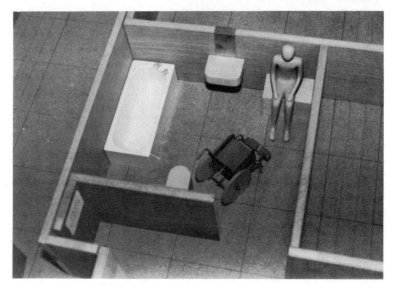

(c)

going for a walk. More seats at strategic points, more shelters where elderly people may wait if they are tired and need to rest, and more effective handrails by steps are needed.

EMPLOYMENT AND OTHER ACTIVITIES

Some occupational therapists will be employed in one or more of a wide range of day and residential establishments run by the local authority, where they will be responsible for activities of a rehabilitative or supportive nature.

Many day centres are based on a model similar to a large department in a hospital or rehabilitation unit. A wide range of individual and group activities will be available, often managed by an occupational therapist. Facilities such as chiropody, bathing, hair dressing and other kinds of individual personal care will be available. Clients may be able to take their washing, ironing or sewing and use the facilities at the day centre. There, with support if required, they can carry out their household activities as independently as possible and return home with a sense of achievement. Meals and other

245

Figure 13.2: Layout plans (a) before and (b) after adaptation

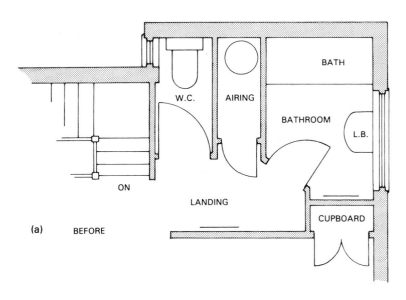

(a)   BEFORE

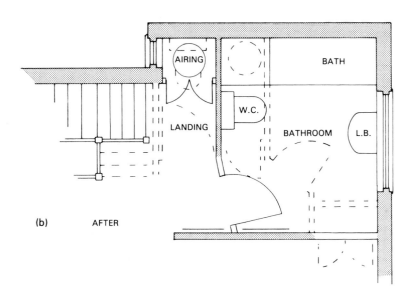

(b)   AFTER

refreshments ensure that clients have at least one hot meal per day in a sociable environment. Many day centres have a small shop which enables those people with more restricted mobility to purchase basic essentials and some small luxuries.

Ideally, there will be a complementary mix of staff and voluntary workers at these centres who will help to provide friendly support for the clients and also participate in care-planning to ensure that clients experience a rich quality of life. Popular activities might, for example, include cookery, painting, pottery, singing, carpentry and horticulture.

Clients may either make their own way to the day centre, obtain a lift from a relative or friend or, particularly if they use a wheelchair and require the tail lift, use the social services transport.

Increasingly, occupational therapists are employed to work in residential or Part III homes. Again, the purpose is to provide a service similar to that which will be found in a good geriatric ward of a hospital, with emphasis on independence, dignity and a good quality of life.

QUALITY

The importance of setting and maintaining high standards is one which is frequently threatened by shortages of suitably trained and qualified staff. A highly-committed occupational therapist will attract other highly-committed staff and students. If the teamwork is good and the atmosphere friendly and efficient, it is likely that students will wish to return once they have become qualified.

Supervision of students and junior staff must be carried out by another professional who is properly trained and up-to-date with current practice. This is particularly important now that the occupational therapy colleges have developed their individual Diploma '81 Courses and require that clinical supervisors are familiar with the specific needs of that course.

Occupational therapists should be managed by senior occupational therapists and, where devolved into patch or area teams, should be coordinated by a principal occupational therapist, working closely with his/her colleagues in the NHS.

The tremendous shortage of qualified occupational therapists in the United Kingdom will not be overcome quickly unless there is a far greater commitment from government to financing additional training places, and to encouraging new initiatives and incentives which will entice those therapists who have left the profession back to work. The profession needs to review the recruitment and selection processes when seeking suitable students. Some research should also be carried out to discover why occupational therapists leave the profession and at what stage. Career counselling and development need to be improved, enabling a greater choice of opportunity for promotion.

It is difficult to know the exact numbers of practising occupational therapists and their distribution. This is due to the use of other titles, such as independent living advisor, and also because not every therapist belongs to the British Association of Occupational Therapists (BAOT). Recent figures obtained from BAOT indicate that in the United Kingdom out of a membership of 8,000, approximately 1,000 occupational therapists work in local authorities.

14

Methods of Record Keeping

Lindsay Winterton and Linda Haldane

Record keeping is important for all patients but has particular advantages when working with the elderly. There are several medical conditions which may result in the patient being disorientated when first seen, or their memory may be affected. This leads to problems in obtaining relevant information perhaps for several days during which effective management is difficult. As elderly patients are frequently re-admitted with either new or recurring problems, records from a previous admission can give valuable background information and a picture of the patient's previous ability. Recording of decisions made, by whom and why a particular course was pursued or discarded may prevent the ground being fruitlessly covered again in the future.

WHY KEEP RECORDS?

There are several reasons why record keeping must be taken as a serious task in patient care. It should provide a method of clearly documenting an elderly patient's problems, management, expected achievements, discharge plans and the effectiveness, or otherwise, of treatment.

In this chapter we examine systems which fulfil these objectives — and mention other considerations to take into account when establishing accurate record keeping.

Legal requirements

In all professions' codes of practice there are clauses covering the confidentiality of information. In the medical professions, such confidentiality is essential with regard to patients' medical notes.

It is also essential for the protection of staff that accurate records are kept as in the event of litigation these records would be acceptable as evidence. In the area of social work records there has been a change of practice over the last five years, in response to pressure from clients — acceded to by the government in 1983 — to allow open access to their files (Data Protection Act 1984).

When passing on information regarding a patient to other members of the multidisciplinary team it is important that they treat the information as confidential.

Communication

Medical records must give an accurate account of the patient's problems, treatment and the state of the patient on discharge. This information should be gathered, and may be used, by all members of the multidisciplinary team caring for the patient, thus providing the core of information for communication.

Education

Records may be used to review process of care and treatment leading to identification of gaps in either services or in professionals' own knowledge. The records are also a useful tool in the teaching of students and junior staff.

Research

The examination of medical records should be able to give accurate data which can be used in research. The type of system used for record keeping makes the auditing of information hard or easy; and not all methods give standardisation of data. Where such standardisation is absent records will be invalid for research.

FAILURE OF PRESENT SYSTEMS

Systems of record keeping are many and, equally, so are failures in systems. We look at five common failures below.

(i) Most of the individual disciplines making up the multi-disciplinary team tend to keep their own separate records, making communication between members very poor.

(ii) After initial assessment, records kept may only present a diary of treatment sessions. They do not include any form of future progression, aims and goals of a patient or projected outcome as a result of treatment given. Daily treatment sessions appear to have little connection with the overall function of the patient.

(iii) There is difficulty in retracing reasoning behind decisions made for patient's care, as medical records are source-orientated, mixing information about all sorts of problems. This makes it unclear what is, or what is not, being done for the patient.

(iv) There is a tendency for staff to treat patients' problems from their own viewpoint rather than that of the patients.

(v) Present systems give no logical method for the abstraction of information for research.

FUTURE SYSTEMS AVAILABLE

There is obviously a need to develop a more organised approach to record keeping, making communication between all disciplines more effective, thus improving the quality of patient care and facilitating the use of treatments shown to be effective. We look at five such systems — POMR, NP, Community Coordinators, Photography and Video Recording, Computer Systems.

POMR (PROBLEM-ORIENTED MEDICAL RECORDS)

The pioneer of POMR as a method of record keeping was Lawrence L. Weed, an American physician. He developed POMR in 1968 and most systems used today are based on Weed's original work (Weed 1968).

Figure 14.1: Patient's problem list, often used as a front sheet to medical records

Diagnosis:	In Patient ☐ Ward: Out Patient ☐ Therapist			
Clinical Details Recent:				
Distant:				
Drugs:	O.T. S.W. Sp Th. HV/DN			
Occupation Current or previous	Home Help ☐ Meals on Wheels ☐ Transport Y/N			

PROBLEM LIST

Number	Active	Date	Resolved/Inactive	Date

Hospital No.

Surname (block letters)

Forename

Address

D of B / /

Tel no.

M/F   M/W/S/D

G.P.

Consultant

Date of next appointment

ADMISSION   DATE OF   DISCHARGE

When used properly by the multidisciplinary team, POMR facilitates quality of care, and clearly defines the role of each discipline in the patient's overall care and treatment aimed at functional independence. For those who use POMR, it demands that they strive for excellence by taking a logical and analytical approach to the care of patients.

In current practice, POMR is used mainly by occupational therapists and physiotherapists. In some elderly persons' units, medical staff do use a patient's problem list (Figure 14.1) as a front sheet to medical records.

There are five main elements in the construction of POMR:

(i) The data base.
(ii) The problem list.
(iii) The initial plan.
(iv) Progress notes.
(v) Discharge summary.

These five elements will be fully explained to include special modifications and additions with regard to documenting the needs of elderly people. (In this explanation of the use of POMR it is assumed that the records will be used by all members of the multidisciplinary team.)

The data base

When used by all members of the multidisciplinary team the complete medical record should have a full list of all the patient's problems. This list should be 'dynamic', being changed and updated at any time. Thus, POMR can be used as an effective form of communication. The members of the team must define each problem (by collecting data), decide on the appropriate treatment and expected outcome, and use a systematic documentation of this outcome. Once a problem has been identified and recorded it cannot be overlooked or forgotten.

Thus, POMR gives team members the means to improve their methods of overall assessment and it also helps to educate junior staff in the needs of the elderly patient.

Collection of data will form the data base, which consists of all information about the patient collected by all members of the multidisciplinary team and entered in the records. This information is subjective and objective:

— personal data (e.g. name, age, address, etc.)
— medical history, physical examination, drugs and laboratory results
— social history and situation, community support and accommodation
— names of the members of the multidisciplinary team
— provisional diagnosis

The above are statutory for an accurate data base, but it is also possible to include additional functional abilities, activities of daily living, faecal and urinary incontinence — all in the form of assessment charts.

The problem list

From the information collected in the data base it becomes possible for the team to draw up a list of the patient's problems. Each problem is numbered and it is essential to date each problem as it is charted on the records. The problem list has an active and inactive column, problems moving to the inactive column when they become quiescent or solved by any action taken.

At a quick glance, it should be possible to immediately ascertain the patient's problems as an individual.

The initial plan

An individual patient care and treatment programme is made for each of the patient's numbered problems. The care programme may consist of any medical tests, treatment or action taken by members of the team aiming to solve the problem, in consultation with the patient.

It is easy to establish the role of each discipline in the patient's management, and demands that careful thought and logical action is made, ensuring that everyone, including the patient, is working towards an agreed objective.

Progress notes

It is only necessary to write any progress notes when there has been change and need for new information to be recorded. Each progress note relates to a specific problem and is numbered and written under four headings: subjective, objective, assessment and plan. Progress notes are often referred to, utilising their initials, as SOAP notes. These need further clarification.

Subjective The SOAP notes (Figure 14.2) will contain information stated by the patient about his problem. In the elderly population, where patients may have an altered mental state (e.g. confusional state, disorientation, poor short-term memory) it is often necessary to state information given by carers as long as the source of information is clear.

Objective The multidisciplinary team's observations and changes in signs are recorded here. They can include clinical recordings, functional ability, ADL, etc. As the SOAP notes continue, the objective heading is therefore used to record reassessment of the patient.

Assessment This is the evaluation of the information recorded in the subjective and objective findings, allowing the team to identify long- and short-term goals to solve the patient's problems. Good use of assessment heading ensures that the disciplines are thinking logically and realistically about their patient's problems and treatment plans.

Plan Shows the way in which the treatment plans are developed to achieve the goals set (e.g. the frequency of treatment by therapists). The plan obviously needs to be updated and changed if either no progress is made and the treatment is of no effect; or if the improvement necessitates changes in level or approach. We also need to take into consideration necessary changes in the plan if the patient's general condition or situation changes.

Progress notes only need to be charted if there has been any change. It is essential that each addition is dated and initialled by the writer to identify source of information. It is not necessary to record information under S, O, A and P on each entry but only that which is relevant. However, each heading should be accompanied by a problem number.

255

Figure 14.2: Example of SOAP note

Date	No.	SOAP	Patient's Name ....BROWN..............	Initial
26457	②	S O A P	Feeling better. Pain in R hip much less R side Walked 10 yds in Kaut limping Pain settling in lk require analgesics Cont bed xs, Transfer practice Increase walking activity on ward	LH

Discharge summary

When the patient is discharged from the care of the team, the discharge summary should give an up-to-date picture in relation to the original problem list. The summary should briefly state how problems were resolved, and explain why some problems may be continuing and how they can be managed in the future. A good summary gives an accurate picture of the patient's condition and capabilities at the time of discharge. It is also a good baseline from which to start if the patient is re-admitted at some future date. Again, a date and legible signature is essential.

There may be additional headings, such as for 'MDT meetings' (multidisciplinary team), to record information quickly and effectively, keeping developments towards possible discharge up-to-date. In order to make the source of information clear, there may be a use of a different colour ink for each discipline.

Advantages of POMR

At first glance the use of POMR looks a very time-consuming form of record keeping. However, SOAP notes are never written unless there is a new or additional data to record. Therefore, it can be assumed that the last SOAP note recorded is the most up-to-date information on a patient's problem. This can cause problems when treating elderly people who, for reasons of forgetfulness or manipulation, claim they have not had treatment. A perpetual calendar on the front sheet with the days of treatment given and crossed through as they are completed may help — or, alternatively, something found to record under S, O, A or P.

When used by all team members the records will provide documentation of the health care given to the patient as a whole person functioning in daily life. POMR provides documented evidence as to whether or not the treatment is beneficial to the patient, making needs to change treatments more apparent.

The disciplines using POMR are encouraged to state professional opinions on the patient's progress, a factor generally avoided. Such a method of record keeping used by all members of the team must result in better communication and, therefore, promote better quality of individual patient care. In turn this must result in a higher turnover of hospital beds, as demonstrated in the implementation of a similar in-patient records system at a rehabilitation hospital for the elderly (Rosenburg *et al.* 1986).

In conclusion, each patient should have a single medical document, recording all his medical and social problems and their treatment given in hospital or out-patient care and at home.

POMR can fulfil this need.

THE NURSING PROCESS

POMR may be used by one discipline alone or by several together. An ideal development of this, as we have seen in Chapter 7, is the Nursing Process (NP). Usually it is initially developed by the nursing staff but when established all the members of the multidisciplinary team may have an input into the recording system.

They may also obtain a large amount of data for their own needs from that recorded by the nurse. This is an advantage for the patient as he is not being repeatedly asked for the same basic information by several people in succession. It is important that the patient is told that information given to the internal interviewer may be passed on to other members of the team. Members, too, may write directly into the nursing notes (using a different colour ink for each discipline), or there may be a separate sheet within the NP for non-nursing staff to enter information.

There is a planned systematic approach to the care of the individual patient. Nursing care in the past has often been disease-related. In the NP it is linked to ADL. Roper *et al.* (1985) lists these as:

— maintaining a safe environment
— communicating
— breathing
— eating and drinking
— elimination of body wastes
— personal cleansing and dressing
— controlling body temperature
— mobilising
— working and playing
— expressing sexuality
— sleeping
— dying

This may mean a change of emphasis in the way in which nurses work as well as the method of recording. Previously, for many nurses, the work has been very much task-orientated (e.g. washing, bathing, dressing of wounds, ulcers to be done) and care has been allocated on task lines, one nurse carrying out all the dressings to be done on the ward whilst another was given a list of patients to be helped with bathing and so on. This means that each patient could have several nurses caring for him in the space of one morning.

With the NP each nurse is responsible for a group of patients, attending to all their nursing needs on an individual basis.

Operation of NP

Operation of the nursing process has four elements:

- (i) Assessment including data collection.
- (ii) Planning.
- (iii) Implementation.
- (iv) Evaluation.

Assessment The assessment is carried out with the patient and/or his family in order to identify problems. Together they agree on objectives and decide the care needed for each problem (the Care Plan). During assessment not only current problems are considered but also potential ones; thus prevention is also part of the planning. Included in the initial assessment is collection of data including nursing and social information, why the patient thinks he was admitted to hospital, his usual pattern of daily life and so on.

Regular re-assessment and appropriate modification of the Care Plan are carried out as needs change.

Planning Planning will include goal-setting and the plans by which these goals can be achieved, taking into account the physical environment plus equipment and nursing time available. For instance, it would be preferable for the patient to maintain his mobility by walking to the bathroom; this can be achieved with the aid of two nurses but will there be two nurses available all the time? If this is unlikely then the goal set is unrealistic.

Goals should be both short- and long-term. Short-term could be walking to the bathroom with one nurse within one week if at present he needs the help of two people. The long-term goal for the same problem may be walking without the assistance of another person but perhaps with some form of walking aid.

Plans should relate to specific problems or potential problems; the action to be taken should be recorded in sufficient detail to enable another person taking over the patient's care to provide continuity of care.

Implementation The Care Plan may not always be 'doing' but could include observations of a patient's behaviour (e.g. whether he eats all his meal). It could be making sure that the environment is appropriate for the patient to achieve the goal set (e.g. making sure he can reach his clothes in order to dress himself by placing the locker in a convenient position).

Evaluation The last phase of the NP is evaluation. The nurse decides if goals have been met. If not, she needs to consider why not and to formulate new plans to solve the problem. If the goals have been achieved, the next stage for which a goal needs to be set, and a plan to achieve it, must be decided.

Though NP may initially be used only by nursing staff it can be used to include all problems, goals and actions identified and agreed by the multidisciplinary team.

COMMUNITY CO-ORDINATORS

One of the problems in caring for elderly people in the community is the exchange of information between possibly several people providing varied and sometimes overlapping services. Often personal or telephone contact is used, particularly if there is need for discussion, but this assumes that the two people concerned know of the involvement of each other — but this is not always so.

One method of ensuring that everyone involved knows of the existence of others is a surveillance card. One such example has been fully described elsewhere (Pearlgood 1987). It contains a general picture of the patient and all the professionals involved, current medication, with room for a date and action taken by the individuals concerned, and contact dates. This is kept in a centrally located filing box for ease of access.

If the district nurse is visiting she will usually keep her case notes in an envelope in the patient's home. On the outside of the envelope will be details of how to contact the district nurse or GP in case of need. The nurse will often leave the date of her next planned visit.

Another record which the patient may have is a medication card (Figure 14.3). If kept up to date this is helpful both to the patient and to the professional visiting. Problems may arise if the card becomes out of date and contains incorrect information or if the patient forgets to produce the card at the right time. Some such cards

Figure 14.3: An example of a medication card as designed and used in Riverside Health Authority, London

MEDICATION CARD

Patient's Name ....

Address ....

Hospital Number .... Tel. ....

Family Doctor .... Tel. ....

Always bring this card and your medicines with you on each visit to the hospital.

Card issued by: Pharmacy Department
St Mary Abbots Hospital, Marloes Road
Kensington W8 5LQ.
Tel. 01-937 8181 Ext. 536

		Breakfast time	Lunch time	Evening meal	Bed time

have room for a sample of the drug to be taken to be fixed to the card as a reminder to the patient as to what to take when.

All these records have value but also pitfalls so that care always needs to be taken when using them (Weed 1971). The majority do not record the lay help provided and this may be a useful addition, and should always be enquired about.

PHOTOGRAPHY AND VIDEO RECORDING

Still photography has been used for many years to record such things as the posture of a patient before and after treatment, or varicose ulcers showing progress before, during and after treatment. A photograph can give a much clearer picture and provide an easier method of comparison than can a multitude of words.

Video recording, as well as providing a record, can be used as an educational tool with the patient. For instance, he can see and, with help, analyse his walking pattern and see at which points he needs to make changes.

COMPUTER SYSTEMS

Computers are likely to be used in the future for the keeping of patients' records. At present POMR and NP are accomplished by manually structured methods. The most obvious way forward in coping with this information overload is to computerise these systems. Both POMR and NP provide the ideal structure for entry onto a computer system, but first it would be necessary for all the members of the multidisciplinary team to establish a well-defined standardised, notation system.

SUMMARY

There seems to be no standardisation of record keeping in any of the professions involved in care of the elderly. The use of POMR and NP by the multidisciplinary team may provide two methods of overcoming the problem of communication to give good all-round quality care to the elderly person. However, there is the problem of standardisation even when these two systems still exist.

Good practice in methods of record keeping in the future should follow along the lines of POMR and NP in association with the use of computer systems.

REFERENCES

Data Protection Act (1984) HMSO, London

Pearlgood, M. (1987) Surveillance card to help keep an eye on the elderly. *Geriatric Medicine, 17*, 2, 78–9

Roper, N., Logan, W.W. and Tierney, A.J. (1985) *The Elements of Nursing*. Churchill Livingstone, Edinburgh

Rosenburg, W., Parkes, J., Jenkins, A., Denham, M., Royston, J.P., Sullens, C.M., O'Neil, C. and Dobbs, S.M. (1986) Making a rehabilitation hospital for the elderly work. *Health Trends, 18*, 66–71

Weed, L. (1968) Medical records that guide and teach. *New England Journal of Medicine* (March), 593–600

———— (1971) Quality control and the medical record. *Archive of International Medicine, 127*, 101–5

Appendix I

Alison Froggatt

(a) *National Assistance Act (1948), Part III, Section 21,*
Residential Accommodation
A local authority may provide residential accommodation for persons
who 'by reasons of age are in need of care and attention which is
not otherwise available to them'. This is Part III of the Act, and
hence the colloquial and widely used shorthand of 'Part III' to refer
to local authority residential homes.

(b) *National Assistance Act (1948) as amended Section 47*
Adults can be placed in institutional care for the necessary care and
attention if they are suffering from grave chronic disease, or being
aged, are infirm, physically incapacitated, and living in insanitary
conditions. Secondly, it must be shown that they are unable to look
after themselves, and are not receiving proper care and attention
from others.

This Act which involves taking away a person's liberty, on the
recommendation of the community physician, and consent of a
magistrate, is much disputed, and irregularly used. (For a fuller
discussion see Age Concern 1986.)

(c) *Health Services and Public Health Act (1968), Section 45*
Under this Act the local authority is empowered to carry out many
of the major services for the welfare of old people, such as Meals-
on-Wheels, boarding out (fostering) elderly people, advice, information, and social work support, warden services, aids and adaptations
in the home, and bus passes. This Act does not give a clear entitlement to these services; their provision in any particular case rests on
there being sufficient resources available.

264

(d) Chronically Sick and Disabled Persons Act (1970)
This Act applies to old people, as it lays a duty on local authorities to inform themselves of the number of old people in the area who come into the categories (under National Assistance Act (1948) Section 29) of being blind, deaf, dumb, suffering from mental disorder, or being substantially and permanently handicapped by illness, injury, congenital deformity, or other such disabilities. The Act identifies certain provisions which would be helpful.

(e) National Health Service Act (1977) Schedule 8
Here local authorities are placed under a duty to provide home helps for households where such help is required by reason of the presence of a person who is aged.

(f) Mental Health Act (1983)
This allows for the provision of Guardianship to a person whose behaviour is confused or bizarre, under Section 7–10. Section 117 creates a duty to provide an after-care for people mentally ill.

(g) Registered Homes Act (1984)
Regulations to register and inspect residential care homes for four or more people, run privately. The Act contains guidance only, with more detail in *Home Life* (Centre for Policy on Ageing 1984).

(h) Powers of Attorney Act 1971. Enduring Powers of Attorney Act 1985
These two Acts are to protect the affairs of someone aware of becoming mentally incapacitated, by appointing an attorney to Act for him/her. A full discussion of the different provisions of the Acts can be found in the Age Concern publication on legal matters (Age Concern 1986).

Despite these Acts: 'Social service departments have very few statutory responsibilities towards elderly people, a few powers to protect, none to represent them, and limited resources to help. This is often overlooked when tragic situations are given extensive media coverage' (Age Concern 1986).

(i) Disabled Persons (Services, Consultation and Representation) Act 1986
This Act allows for authorised representatives of disabled persons to be appointed. The local authority has a duty to take into account the abilities of a carer when deciding about the provision of services.

REFERENCES

Age Concern (1986) *The Law and Vulnerable Elderly People*. Age Concern, Mitcham, 34, 39–49

Centre for Policy on Ageing (1984) *Home Life*. Centre for Policy on Ageing, London

The following publications referred to in the text may be obtained from HMSO bookshops:

The Chronically Sick and Disabled Persons Act 1970, pp. 1, 8

1976 Amendment to the Chronically Sick and Disabled Persons Act, p. 17

The Disabled Persons (Services, Consultation and Representation) Act 1986, pp. 2, 3, 7, 8, 17

Data Protection Act 1984, p. 5

Disabled Persons Act 1981, p. 17

Appendix II

Alison Froggatt

Tom, aged 73, lived alone as a widower in a small rented cottage. He had had one leg amputated for gangrene following peripheral vascular disease but returned home to cope quite well. His only daughter visited regularly. A stroke 18 months later, followed by a second amputation, changed the picture. As he was mentally alert and friendly, it was hoped he could be rehabilitated to use a wheelchair and become fit enough for an old peoples' home. The social worker was involved in discussing these suggestions with him, being aware of all the losses he had already experienced. It was necessary to intervene with the landlady, at his request, as she wanted to give him notice to quit, and to work closely with the daughter too. The time waiting for a vacancy was usefully spent not only in physical rehabilitation but also in grief work, helping him to come to terms with all that had happened, so that he was more ready for a new start when the time came.

An elderly lady, Amy, lived alone in a rented flat. She burnt her hands when pieces of newspaper supplements fell out onto her electric fire. She could not return to the flat. Her social worker did considerable work with her about the losses in her life, of her possessions, and flat, and rescued a deed box which was particularly precious. Her future care could not be discussed until this work was done. Amy improved well and wanted to go to sheltered housing, rather than an old peoples' home. A flat was obtained but needed redecoration, and because of pressure on beds the old lady was moved to a convalescent home for two weeks. As the flat was still not ready she had a week in a private old peoples' home. When the day came to go to her new flat she refused to go, and had by then decided the small private rest home suited her needs very well. This work took a good deal of time, and effort with many contacts with the few relatives and neighbours, and with outside agencies. In the end, respecting the old lady's wishes as far as possible at each stage, Amy and the social worker were left feeling she had made the right decision about the level of care and independence she wanted, following her burn injury and rehabilitation in hospital.

Appendix III

Useful Addresses

Age Concern
Bernard Sunley House, 60
  Pitcairn Road
Mitcham, Surrey
CR4 3LL

Alzheimer's Disease Society
Bank Buildings, Fulham
  Broadway
London SW16 1EP

Association of Carers
Medway Homes, Balfour Road
Rochester, Kent

Association of Continence
  Advisors
c/o Disabled Living Foundation
380–384 Harrow Road
London W9 2HU

Association of Professional Music
  Therapists
c/o 76 Gosport Road
London

Bedside Manners
Highgate New Town Community
  Centre
25 Bertram Street
London N19 5DQ

A company of theatrical actors

specialising in bringing plays
to hospitals, day centres, old
people's homes, etc.

British Association of
  Occupational Therapists
20 Rede Place
London W2 4TU

British Diabetic Association
10 Queen Anne Street
London W1M 0BD

Centre on Environment for the
  Handicapped
35 Great Smith Street
London SW1P 3BJ

Centre for Policy on Ageing
25–31 Ironmonger Row
London EC1V 3QP

The College of Occupational
  Therapists
20 Rede Place
Bayswater
London W2 4TU

Chest, Heart & Stroke
  Association
Tavistock House North, Tavistock
  Square
London WC1H 9JE

269

Commission for Racial Equality
10–12 Allington Street
London SW1E 5EH

The Disabled Living Foundation
380–384 Harrow Road
London W9 2HU

Health Education Council
78 New Oxford Street
London WC1A 1AH

Help the Aged
St James Walk
London EC1R 0BE

Kings Fund Centre
126 Albert Street
London NW1 7NF

MIND
22 Harley Street
London W1N 2ED

National Extension College
18 Brooklands Avenue
Cambridge CB2 2HN

Royal Association for Disability
and Rehabilitation
25 Mortimer Street
London W1N 8AB

Winslow Press
Telford Road
Bicester, Oxfordshire
OX6 0TS
Produce excellent visual aids for
use with those patients
overcoming orientation
problems

Index

Page references in *italics* refer to Figures or Tables.